W9-APN-933

ADVANCE PRAISE FOR

FIT CITIES

"This public health crusader's gripping narrative is essential reading for policymakers, practitioners, and anyone genuinely curious about what actually makes us healthy." —Lawrence Loh, Associate Medical Officer of Health for Peel Region and Adjunct Professor at Dalla Lana School of Public Health at the University of Toronto

"Dr. Lee retraces key developments in our understanding of the importance of our life and work environments in preventing obesity, diabetes, cardiovascular diseases, and cancers through her work with health departments in the United States, Colombia, Canada, Australia, Singapore, and the United Kingdom. Her professional journey reflects the global challenge of modifying the settings we live and work in to reverse lifestyle risk factors associated with non-communicable diseases. From reducing unhealthy food consumption to increasing physical activity and developing holistic approaches to promoting healthy living 'as a default,' her account provides insightful glimpses into the challenges, constraints, solutions, and achievements of public health and policy." —Yoong Kang Zee, CEO, Health Promotion Board, Singapore

"This book is a must-read for anyone who wants to know why we aren't making progress in preventing chronic diseases like hypertension and diabetes. Dr. Karen Lee exposes how today's environment is fighting against our efforts to optimally manage chronic diseases and their risk factors like obesity. She weaves intriguing real-life stories of how simple interventions can create health. Care providers and patients alike should take note!" —Dr. Nadia Khan, MD, FRCPC, Professor and Interim Head of General Internal Medicine Division, University of British Columbia; President, Hypertension Canada; co-author, Diabetes Canada Guidelines

"Designing for health is one of the most urgent issues of our time. In this book, Dr. Karen Lee, leading protagonist of the Active Design Movement, charts the course of her own personal vision and journey and not only clearly establishes that human health is influenced by the physical and social environments in which we live and work, but also demonstrates what can be accomplished with true dedication, creative thinking, and above all, cooperation. A must-read for city makers, politicians, urban planners and designers, and for anybody interested in making healthy life choices." —Professor Ben van Berkel, Founder/Principal Architect UNStudio, Amsterdam; Founder UNSense

"*Fit Cities* shows us that some of the world's leading health challenges can be successfully addressed by building key partnerships and bringing inspirational professionals together. City builders, all levels of government, and citizens alike can learn from Dr. Lee's experience, advice, and passion for all of us to achieve healthier outcomes in our professional practice, communities, and personal lives." —Eleanor Mohammed, President, Canadian Institute of Planners (2016–2020) and Deputy Chief Administrative Officer, City of Beaumont

"On-the-ground, in-the-neighbourhood knowledge from a health expert who knows how critical places and spaces are to living our best lives." —Charles Branas, Chair of Epidemiology at Columbia University and co-author of *Changing Places, The Science and Art of New Urban Planning*

"Karen Lee's remarkable career has been devoted to discovering what works for the built environment and health, and the tremendous benefits for health (and quality of life, environmental protection, and improved economic prosperity) to be gained. The richness of the examples she provides from around the world adds to the persuasiveness of her argument for a transformation of our communities from the trend of car-domination we have followed for the best part of a century. *Fit Cities* is an amazing and moving journey." —Dr. Charles Gardner, MD, CCFP, MHSc, FRCPC, Medical Officer of Health and Chief Executive Officer, Simcoe Muskoka District Health Unit, Canada

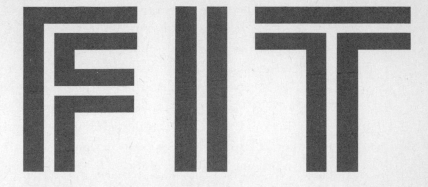

FIT CITIES

My Quest to Improve the World's Health and Wellness— Including Yours

KAREN K. LEE, MD

Doubleday Canada

Copyright © 2020 Karen Lee

All rights reserved. The use of any part of this publication, reproduced, transmitted in any form or by any means electronic, mechanical, photocopying, recording or otherwise, or stored in a retrieval system without the prior written consent of the publisher—or in the case of photocopying or other reprographic copying, license from the Canadian Copyright Licensing agency—is an infringement of the copyright law.

Doubleday Canada and colophon are registered trademarks of Penguin Random House Canada Limited

Library and Archives Canada Cataloguing in Publication

Title: Fit cities : my quest to improve the world's health and wellness—including yours / Karen K. Lee.
Names: Lee, Karen K., author.
Identifiers: Canadiana (print) 20190149566 | Canadiana (ebook) 20190149620 | ISBN 9780385685320 (hardcover) | ISBN 9780385685337 (EPUB)
Subjects: LCSH: Public health. | LCSH: Health. | LCSH: Medicine, Preventive.
Classification: LCC RA425 .L44 2020 | DDC 362.1—dc23

Cover and book design by Leah Springate
Cover images by Yapanda/Getty Images

Printed and bound in Canada

Published in Canada by Doubleday Canada,
a division of Penguin Random House Canada Limited

www.penguinrandomhouse.ca

10 9 8 7 6 5 4 3 2 1

Penguin
Random House
DOUBLEDAY CANADA

To my parents, Andrew Seng-Lok Lee and Anne Liang-Sim Lee,
whose unwavering support and love have given me
fortitude and courage to pursue my dreams.

And to Matthew Lee, Rebecca Lee, and Alysa Englehardt,
that you too will be blessed with the intersection of
serendipity and opportunities from hard work.
As you reach for the stars, may you land there or on the moon.

"Courage is the price that life exacts for granting peace."

—AMELIA EARHART

CONTENTS

NOT YOUR TYPICAL HEALTH BOOK

A NOTE FROM THE AUTHOR

THIS IS NOT a typical health book. You won't find diet advice in these pages, or tips about exercise, supplements, or gut microbes. There isn't a yoga sequence in sight. And you won't read a word about meditation, or the relative dangers of fat, sugar, and salt.

If that's what you're looking for, you're in the wrong place. But before you put this book back on the shelf and go in search of something that has 365 smoothie recipes, I'd ask you to reconsider. This *is* a book about health. It's about your health, and the health of the city or town in which you live. Because—make no mistake—the two are intimately connected.

All too often, health is considered to be a personal responsibility. In countless books and articles about diet and exercise, in countless television show segments dedicated to weight loss, we're told what we need to change in order to achieve better health. But many of us already know these things. In fact, one of health education's major successes over the last several decades is this widespread awareness of the need to modify our behavior. We know what we need to do. Year in and year out, our top New Year's resolutions are weight loss, more exercise, and healthier eating.

But for many of us, it makes no difference. Year in and year out, we are getting fatter.

What's going on?

To answer that question, we need to think about those New Year's resolutions again. The whole idea of a resolution is to *resolve*—to decide firmly on a course of action. We must *resolve* to make changes. We must *choose* to do whatever is in our power to do in order to succeed. As it turns out, that last part is the key: *whatever is in our power to do.* All of our heartfelt and determined resolutions to lose weight, eat better, and exercise more come with a subtle built-in assumption: we can lose weight *if we choose,* eat better *if we choose,* and exercise more *if we choose.* But what if we can't make that choice? What if that's not within our power? We can only make healthy choices around eating if stores and restaurants near our homes have healthy items on offer. We can only walk to work if the sidewalks are in good condition—or there at all. We can only encourage our children to get outside and kick a ball around if there's a safe playground or park nearby.

The commonly held assumption that weight loss is a battle that must be fought alone has caused us to fail miserably in our fight against obesity. Rates of overweight and obesity around the world continue to skyrocket, along with related conditions, because we continue to place blame solely on the individual rather than on the environment in which they live. We continue to prioritize willpower and stick-to-itiveness over access to healthy food. We continue to stress the importance of exercise over the importance of creating opportunities for active living in the places where we spend most of our time.

If we want to reverse the trends of the last several decades, we need to start a new conversation—one that's radically different from what we've been hearing on the news and reading in the pages of books and magazines. We need to talk about what society—the collective *we*—can do better. We need to talk about how to create environments that will help rather than hinder our quest to become healthier.

I don't just believe this, I know it. Nearly a decade and a half has passed since I started helping cities and organizations to improve the environments in which we live, work, and play. I've worked in public health departments in Edmonton, Alberta, and New York City. I've led a team of U.S. Centers for Disease Control and Prevention (CDC) "disease detectives" in a ground-breaking field study into an obesity "outbreak." I've traveled to Bogotá and Singapore, to Sydney and São Paulo, to the U.K. and the Netherlands, among many other places, to consult and learn. Through it all, one thing has become abundantly clear: our success in being healthy depends not only on ourselves—though we certainly have important roles to play and choices to make—but also on the physical and social environments we create in our cities, communities, and organizations. If our cities and towns become fit and healthy, we will find it easier to become fit and healthy too.

So, no, this is not a typical health book. But it just might be the one we all need.

— Dr. Karen Lee

INTRODUCTION

A NEW CONVERSATION

APRIL 24, 2005. More than a decade later, I can still remember how it felt to touch down at Yeager Airport in Charleston, West Virginia. It was a sunny Sunday afternoon, and I was beyond tired. The week leading up to the flight had been a hectic blur—and the six months prior to that hadn't been any easier. Meetings and phone calls and email exchanges. Countless late nights designing and redesigning documents and tools. Shopping expeditions for clipboards and clicker-counters and computer software. Not to mention packing and repacking heavy cases, trying desperately to make everything fit. But finally we were here: a team of "disease detectives" sent by the U.S. Centers for Disease Control and Prevention (CDC) to investigate the state's obesity outbreak.

Yes . . . you read that right. The world's foremost organization in the fight against the spread of infectious diseases—frightening, highly contagious illnesses such as Ebola and Zika—had sent a group of public health professionals into West Virginia to study overweight people. Okay, so that's not entirely accurate. What the CDC was interested in—what *I* was interested in—were the circumstances behind the state's shockingly high rates of a non-contagious disease: obesity. In 2004, West Virginia ranked third among U.S. states for obesity and first for one of obesity's consequences: hypertension, or high blood pressure. The state also ranked second for diabetes, another health condition associated with obesity. More than 10 percent of adults in West Virginia had diabetes at that time, compared to about 6 percent in the rest of the country. An epidemic—also called an "outbreak"—is defined as "rates of disease above expected or normal levels." Based on those parameters, West Virginia was indeed suffering from outbreaks of obesity, diabetes, and hypertension, even when compared to the already high rates of these conditions in the rest of the United States. The question was: Why?

To understand what I was doing in West Virginia—and the importance of the unprecedented work my team was about to tackle—we need to detour into the past.

Once upon a time, I planned on being a doctor—the kind who wore a white coat and carried a stethoscope and spent her days seeing patients. Becoming an expert in the ways our built environment can affect our health wasn't something I envisioned. I never thought I'd spend my working days (and nights, and weekends!) helping cities and organizations around the world become better at supporting healthy lifestyles. Who could dream that up?

I owe this career to a crisis of conscience I experienced between my first and second years of medical school. Sitting on a park bench one warm, breezeless evening, watching the sky melt into an orange-pink sunset, images of my future flashed before my eyes, depressing by contrast: day after day in a clinic or hospital, white walls and gray doors all around, white fluorescent lights above, white doctor's coat hanging to my knees. Instead of excitement at the prospect of being a doctor, I was filled with dread and despair. As much as I liked helping people, it depressed me to think of spending all my days within dreary hospital settings, trying to treat patients suffering from diseases that are largely avoidable in the first place. I sat on that bench until the sky turned dark. The next morning, I made an appointment with the dean of Student Affairs and arranged to take a year off. I knew that conventional medicine wasn't for me; I needed some time to figure out what was.

During that year, I spent a lot of time contemplating the purpose of medicine. I grappled with the question of how a doctor could find meaning in his or her work, especially in cases where no cure was possible. Could meaning be found in helping a patient to face death and face it well, to die in peace? I thought perhaps it could, and I began to think about oncology as a possible specialty. Once again I found myself sitting outside the dean's office, this time with the summer electives catalog on my lap. I was intent on looking up radiation oncology, but a serendipitous thing happened when I opened the book. Instead of landing at the beginning of the *R*s, I ended up near the end of the *P*s—the public health page.

Back then, like many other people, I had no idea what public health even was. Certainly, I had no clue that public health existed as a specialty for physicians. But as I ran my eyes down the page, I became fascinated with the range of work in the field: food safety and restaurant inspections; daycare inspections; water safety and sanitation monitoring; pest control (from controlling mosquitoes that could spread West Nile virus to controlling rabies in raccoons); needle exchange to prevent the spread of HIV and other blood-borne diseases such as Hepatitis B and C; outbreak detection and control; vaccination programs. I signed up.

That summer—and in the years of study and training that followed—I discovered that I loved public health. Because of the good work done in this field, almost all of us can now access safe drinking water simply by turning on our taps. We have programs that provide free treatment to anyone who has contracted tuberculosis or a sexually transmitted infection, in order to prevent the spread to others. Patients who have difficulty following directions on medications for treating tuberculosis are even visited and assisted by public health nurses, ensuring that their illness is treated fully and that antibiotic resistance does not become an issue with our most deadly infectious diseases. And we can monitor these diseases in all of our communities, helping to detect emerging outbreaks and stop them quickly.

Public health, while firmly grounded in science, is also about creativity and innovation—a combination that appealed to the young medical student I was, and still appeals to me today. An example: In 1854, the Soho district of London was in the grip of a deadly cholera outbreak. At the time, the medical profession believed the disease was caused by "miasma," a cloud of infected air that rose from garbage and sewage piles. Dr. John Snow wasn't convinced. He thought that cholera's severe diarrhea might be caused by something people ingested, and that it was possibly passed along not through a cloud of toxic air but through traces of infected feces.

The outbreak gave Snow a chance to test his theory. He visited affected neighborhoods and knocked on doors, questions at the ready: How many people in the house have fallen ill? How many have died? Where do you get your water? Slowly, painstakingly, he mapped the outbreak—and the information he gathered led him to a water pump on Broad Street. It is said that Snow stomped over to the pump and yanked off the handle. With or without that dramatic flourish, his approach worked. The outbreak stopped. At a time when society had few effective ideas regarding how to control infectious diseases, John Snow—the "father of epidemiology"—studied the problem and then implemented a solution based on outside-the-box thinking.

Snow's water pump moment was a decisive victory in the fight against infectious diseases. Around the world, cities took note and began implementing important changes to address sanitation, water and food supply, and living conditions (from overcrowding to proper ventilation and light). New zoning requirements allowed sunlight in to dry out previously perpetual puddles and damp streets that bred disease-carrying mosquitoes. Swamps were drained. Pest control became a priority. The results were dramatic. From the middle of the nineteenth century to the early twentieth century, deaths from infectious diseases like cholera and tuberculosis dropped significantly. With the introduction of vaccines, like those for smallpox and measles, and the creation of programs that provided easy access to them for little or no cost, infectious disease rates dropped even more dramatically. People began to live longer lives.

I loved these "success stories," and I was inspired by the comprehensive, environmentally grounded, systems-based approach that public health brought to the practice of medicine. I loved the idea that there was a "common good," and the notion that it made sense for governments and health organizations to intervene in order to ensure that people had the support they needed to stay healthy and safe. I loved that when these interventions worked, people didn't have to get sick in the first place, and those who were sick could be helped. This was the meaning I'd been looking for during my year off. I'd found it in the study of public health, and I looked forward to applying the discipline's models to the health challenges of our times.

It's hard to believe from today's vantage point, but there was a time when obesity wasn't considered to be the health crisis it is today. Although it had been identified as a key risk factor for cardiovascular diseases in the 1960s, U.S. data from that era suggested that obesity occurred in only a very small percentage of the population. Very few people had a body mass index (BMI)— or weight-to-height ratio—of 30 or higher, the level at which one was considered to be obese. In the 1980s, that would change. That was the decade in which we'd realize just how quickly rates of obesity—and with them, cases of diabetes—were rising.

One of the first to discover this was Dr. Bill Dietz. In 1970, Dietz graduated from the University of Pennsylvania with a medical degree and became a pediatrician, training in Syracuse, New York. He eventually made his way to Boston, earning a PhD in nutritional biochemistry from the Massachusetts Institute of Technology in 1981. Soon after his training ended, Dietz's reputation as an expert on obesity—particularly childhood obesity— took off. In the 1980s, he began documenting the rapid rise in childhood obesity rates in the United States. From his published research, we would learn that by the late 1970s, the condition of being overweight had increased by 39 percent for those between twelve and seventeen years old, and "superobesity" (the term used by Dietz for what we call childhood "obesity" today) had increased by 64 percent. We would learn that the situation was even worse among younger children, with overweight increasing by 54 percent and superobesity by a staggering 98 percent since the 1960s for those aged between six and eleven. In 1984, Dietz's research showed that obesity rates had seasonal and regional differences. And in 1985, he published the first study showing the links between television watching and obesity in children. TV viewing, it would turn out, promoted sedentariness and inactivity as well as unhealthy diets. Unhealthy food consumption— kids stuffing their mouths with chips, cookies, and popcorn as they sat on the couch—was a big part of the dietary issue, but children who watched a significant amount of TV were also watching more food advertising, which would push them to nag their parents for the unhealthy but tantalizing items they had seen on their screens. In 1986, Dietz's research showed that once a child was obese, treatment tended not to work. Prevention, he concluded, was the best defense.

Dietz's research stuck with me as I made my way through school. By the late 1990s and early 2000s, as I worked my way through my Master of Health Science degree and residency training in Public Health and Preventive Medicine at the University of Toronto, the obesity epidemic was spiraling out of control. Rates of obesity and overweight had been rising for more than two decades, and there was no end in sight. In both Canada and the United States, obesity had doubled in adults and tripled in children since the 1970s and 1980s. Health care costs associated with obesity and its consequences, particularly type 2 diabetes, were rising rapidly. Obesity urgently needed a solution.

In my brain, something was starting to percolate. Over the years, I had taught myself to think laterally, to use analogies from one field of study to find possible solutions in another. Now I found myself wondering: Was there a link between Dietz's TV-watching kids and the Soho residents who got their water from a contaminated pump back in 1854? Could we apply lessons from our public health successes of the past—successes that had tackled infectious diseases like cholera and tuberculosis by adapting the environment—to modern, non-contagious health problems like obesity? I was determined to find out.

Unfortunately, I wasn't finding much support. All around me, public health professionals were throwing up their hands in the face of ever-worsening obesity and type 2 diabetes statistics. They were at a loss. The health education messages spread through ads, posters, pamphlets, and the media didn't seem to be making a difference, and a general sense of hopelessness had set in. In health department after health department during my residency, I saw few examples of effective work. On several occasions, I even heard colleagues question whether the obesity and diabetes epidemics were their problems to solve. They wondered if perhaps people were just too lazy or lacking in willpower to stick with healthy-living habits. If that was the case, they reasoned, then maybe there was nothing to be done.

Although this wasn't a conclusion I was prepared to accept, I was running out of places to look for allies. At one point, my residency program director suggested I meet with a researcher to discuss my ideas for a thesis project. I was excited at the possibility of finding a kindred spirit, someone who felt as passionately as I did about the potential for finding a solution to the obesity and resulting chronic disease epidemics in the public health successes of the past. But it didn't go as I'd hoped. I presented my ideas, only to have each one shot down. The researcher responded to an approach I thought was particularly promising with, "Even the crackpots are not studying that."

I left the meeting discouraged but not defeated. I held on to Albert Einstein's observation: "Great spirits have always encountered violent opposition from mediocre minds. The mediocre mind is incapable of understanding the man who refuses to bow blindly to conventional prejudices." I knew there was a link between our environment and our increasing levels of obesity, and I knew I wasn't the only one who had noticed. Several studies from the 1990s already showed this. In 2001, the U.S. Community Preventive Services Task Force, convened by the Department of Health and Human Services, conducted and published a review of the studies into how different community actions impacted the risk factors for obesity like physical inactivity. It confirmed that media campaigns alone were not effective in battling our growing waistlines: there was insufficient evidence that they worked.

But the review also revealed something else—something intriguing. Comprehensive community campaigns *were* effective. When we tackled the problem with a holistic approach—coupling those health messages with changes to the environment in which we lived and worked—people seemed better able to alter their health behaviors. In 2005, the same task force would build on those findings, recommending changes to the ways we construct our streets and communities. New scientific evidence had proven that better, more health-conscious design of human-built environments was associated with astonishing increases—between 35 and 161 percent—in regular physical activity. When streets and neighborhoods were designed for people to walk and bicycle, and to do so safely, they walked and bicycled more. When people had access to physical activity facilities, from playgrounds to parks to walking paths, they got more physical activity and maintained healthier weights. When buildings were designed to encourage healthy choices, such as taking the stairs, people embraced the better options.

Finally, the research was converging with my own efforts to take a public health approach to obesity and its consequent chronic diseases. With the task force's recommendations, the public health field was finally ready to consider a comprehensive approach that included addressing the environments in our buildings, streets, and communities that either supported or were barriers to our healthy life choices.

By the time the U.S. Community Preventive Services Task Force released those recommendations in 2005, I was well on my way to making a career out of helping cities and organizations support healthy living.

Following the completion of my medical training in 2001, I left Toronto in search of a more supportive environment and found it in Edmonton, Alberta. Between 2002 and 2004, I worked in the local public health department as a deputy medical officer of health in charge of non-communicable diseases (NCDs). Among my responsibilities was participation on the steering committee of the Countrywide Integrated Non-communicable Diseases Intervention (CINDI) project. This World Health Organization (WHO) demonstration project was exploring what could be done to address our current epidemics of non-communicable diseases in one locale, this time Alberta, Canada. CINDI would end up creating the Alberta Healthy Living Network, convening over 150 organizations in the province: local and provincial public health departments; non-governmental organizations such as the Heart and Stroke Foundation, the Canadian Cancer Society, and the Canadian Diabetes Association; academic institutions; and even those working in and outside the government in education, recreation, and other related fields. These groups—all with different mandates and goals—were expected to work together to reduce key risk factors such as smoking, physical inactivity, and unhealthy diets.

I attended one of the group's first meetings. Roughly twenty of us sat at a large wood-paneled conference table, a breakfast of fruit salad and bran muffins before us, in a windowless white room lit by fluorescent bulbs. In contrast to the drab surroundings, not much livelier than many of the hospital settings I had encountered in medical school, the people themselves were enthusiastic and excited. High hopes were pinned on the project to create change in Alberta. Some of those present had been working for a long time in non-communicable disease prevention. Some spoke of inertia, and of the lack of partnerships and coordination across organizations, all of which were working in their own silos. Others spoke of the need to move beyond health campaigns, which were increasingly showing themselves to be both expensive and insufficient. The first task, we were told, was to make a plan: What could we do together, and how could we do it?

Drawing on past initiatives, the plan we formulated outlined a multipronged approach. This would include providing the public with more information; educating the professionals who could provide support through counseling in health care settings; challenging government and organizational policies to create environments more supportive of health in our communities, workplaces, and schools; and measuring our impacts.

My task was to co-chair the Surveillance, Research, and Evaluation Working Group. Surveillance, in the context of public health, is a term used to describe the monitoring of disease rates, trends, and risk factors using epidemiological methods. Typically, surveillance has been restricted to serious infectious diseases, for which the law actually requires doctors, hospitals, and laboratories to report occurrences to public health departments for tracking. Today, reportable infections include blood-borne diseases such as HIV and Hepatitis B and C; sexually transmitted infections such as gonorrhea, syphilis, and chlamydia (in addition to HIV and Hepatitis B); tuberculosis and influenza; water-borne diseases such as cholera; food-borne diseases such as salmonella and E. coli infection; and animal- and insect-transmitted diseases such as rabies, plague, and Lyme disease. It is through such reporting, and the regular monitoring of disease rates and trends in our communities, that outbreaks of these infections are often identified, ideally early enough to prevent further spread.

Surveillance for non-communicable diseases and their risk factors, on the other hand, is not undertaken in many communities. Although national surveys were being conducted in Canada at that time, and annual state-level surveys were occurring in the United States, the data needed for monitoring NCDs and risk conditions such as tobacco use, obesity, physical inactivity, and poor diets *within communities* was at the time—and still is—largely lacking. I knew we needed to get to work on building this community-level information. It is vital for understanding a community's specific needs, and for determining whether various public health actions are having the desired effect.

We were making good progress in Edmonton, and I loved the creative, cooperative, proactive nature of our work, but an irresistible opportunity was on the horizon. In late 2003, I traveled to Atlanta, Georgia, for an interview with the U.S. Centers for Disease Control and Prevention's Epidemic Intelligence Service (EIS). The EIS is an elite team of scientists, medical doctors, and PhD-level professionals—the "disease detectives"—assembled by the CDC and rotated every two years to all corners of the United States, and even the globe when needed, to investigate disease outbreaks and bring them under control. Formed in 1951, the EIS fights on the frontlines of public health. To date, more than three thousand men and women have been deployed. To highlight the division's field-based nature and focus, the imprint of the sole of a shoe has been used as its symbol; field epidemiology is also called "shoe-leather epidemiology." In many ways, this was my dream job—a chance to work for one of the world's largest and most respected public health organizations, a chance to put all of my training to use.

I remember sitting outside the director's office waiting for my interview and offering up a silent prayer: *Please let me think clearly. Please let my responses be knowledgeable and interesting, yet humble.* It must have worked: a few months later, I learned I was one of roughly a hundred candidates from the United States and around the world to be accepted into the disease detectives program.

On a warm, sunny day in June 2004, with my father along for the ride, I climbed into my black, two-door 1999 Honda and began a five-day drive. We traveled south to Montana through the snow-peaked mountains of Glacier National Park, then through Yellowstone, past its blowing geysers and bison herds. We emerged east of the red mountains of Wyoming and headed for the long stretches of flat plains in South Dakota. We took a short detour to see the four presidents carved into Mount Rushmore— inspiring to two Canadians, and an appropriate preparation for my life in the United States—and then continued to Illinois, where we stopped for our first visit to Chicago, a relief after two days of nothing but dry grass, cattle, and farmhouses on the horizon. Then Nashville, which we were too tired to tour. And, finally, Atlanta.

Hot, humid, sunny weather greeted us. Lush with trees and foliage, Atlanta is a city of about half a million residents located within a metropolitan area of suburban sprawl whose combined communities raise the population to over four million. With my father's help, I quickly found an apartment in the Virginia Highlands area, only a block from Piedmont Park—the beautiful in-town green space designed by the sons of New York's Central Park designer Frederick Law Olmsted, and one of two areas in Atlanta at the time that had walkable streets that would take me to nearby restaurants and even an art-house movie theater. I was thrilled that the apartment complex also had an outdoor swimming pool. My first day of work arrived, my father flew home to Canada, and I headed to the CDC.

Although EIS is a separate program within the CDC, its officers are deployed throughout different divisions. Most work within the Center for Infectious Disease Control, some focusing on improving the prevention and control of long-standing infections such as tuberculosis or sexually transmitted diseases or waterborne diseases still rampant in the developing world. Others work on emerging infections such as new strains of the flu. Still others dedicate themselves to rare but scary diseases like Ebola. Only a handful are assigned to the National Center for Chronic Disease Prevention. This was, in fact, my assignment of choice. I had chosen the Physical Activity and Health Branch within the Division of Nutrition, Physical Activity, and Obesity in order to work on the environmental and policy-change projects they wanted to undertake to boost physical activity and improve obesity and chronic disease rates in the United States.

On that first day, I was shown to my office on the fifth floor of a mid-rise building covered in black reflective glass at CDC's

Koger Campus, one of a number of campuses across Atlanta where CDC located its employees. A small, windowless office sparsely furnished with a desk, computer, phone, and rolling chair would greet me daily from 2004 to 2006. I was eager to get to work, and eager to partner with Drs. William Kohl and Michael Pratt, whom I'd met at a conference a few months earlier. An important factor bound Bill and Mike together, and me with them: we shared a drive for finding creative new ways to help support people—and the local and state health departments that were, in turn, trying to help them—to achieve their health goals around behavior change, obesity, and non-communicable diseases. One of the things I loved most about my time working with the Physical Activity and Health Branch was the sense that we were aligned in our willingness to take risks, to identify or create new solutions grounded in emerging science. We were optimists who believed fervently that if we tried, we could find answers even to seemingly intractable current-day epidemics like obesity and diabetes. For the first time in my life, I felt free to voice my many ideas, including some I'd started exploring as far back as my time in Toronto. I felt appreciated for being creative and innovative. I was not only supported but also encouraged to pursue the ideas that "even the crackpots" were not pursuing. In fact, one of those ideas was about to become a reality.

Like all new CDC EIS recruits, I spent my first month on the job in an intensive EIS course. We learned about our DISC (Dominant, Influential, Steady, Conscientious) personality types, and how important they were to our success as a team. Since many of us had not had formal management training at that point, it was probably the first time that we'd started thinking about how to make our teams more effective with people of different personalities: Dominant people, who could make decisions in the face of uncertainty; Influential people, whose team interactions influenced people positively; Steady people, who would ensure the supports for getting things done well; and Conscientious people, whose constant analyses and quests for data would ensure that details did not get missed. We learned the epidemiology methods and computer programs we'd be using in our work. We did mock field studies to prepare us for the real outbreaks that we'd soon be expected to help investigate and bring under control.

It was at this course that I met Julie Sinclair. Julie was a quiet, soft-spoken brunette with thick, shoulder-length hair, slightly taller than my five foot three, and perhaps a few years older than I was. Julie was in Atlanta for the course but had recently moved to West Virginia for her two-year CDC assignment as their state health department's EIS officer. My ears perked up when I heard that. West Virginia: home to some of the worst obesity rates in the country. Like most EIS officers, Julie was assigned to assist her health department's infectious disease division to better monitor, investigate, and control epidemics. Obesity, hypertension, and diabetes—all non-communicable diseases—weren't in her job description. But I wasn't about to let that stop me. I wanted to get my boots on the ground in West Virginia. I wanted to get up close and personal with the environments in which obesity and its related consequences were thriving. I wanted to answer that all-important question—"Why?"—and the equally important "What can we do about it?" Julie was my "in"—an ally on the ground, if she was willing to help.

She was. In order for the CDC to bring a team to West Virginia, we had to be invited. Julie got it done. She connected me to obesity prevention staff working in the state's Bureau for Public Health. I would soon find out that the timing of that call was perfect. West Virginia was in the midst of developing a plan to address its obesity problem, and it needed more data to determine where it should focus its interventions. Was it schools? Worksites? Community settings like restaurants and grocery stores? And what items in those settings needed to be addressed? Where were the barriers to physical activity and healthy eating? Was the environment supportive of the behavior changes people needed to make to conquer obesity?

Not long after those initial conversations, West Virginia's state health commissioner sent a formal request to the CDC's Epidemic Intelligence Service: Could we please send a team to West Virginia to help investigate the state's obesity "outbreak"? CDC leadership approved the request. The "crackpot idea" was finally in motion.

Our touchdown in Charleston was the culmination of months of hard work. Because we were applying outbreak investigation methods to non-communicable disease conditions, something that had rarely been done before, we needed to reinvent the wheel. We had to find—and in some cases develop—the data collection tools and methods we'd need. Tackling that monumental task with me were epidemiologists Dr. Andrea Sharma and Dr. Michele Maynard, who worked on nutrition issues at the CDC, and Dr. Candace Rutt, the CDC's resident scientist specializing in the built environment and physical activity. Together, we developed the surveys and observational recording forms we would use to assess the healthiness of the environments in West Virginia schools, worksites, restaurants, grocery stores, and convenience stores, and the streets that surrounded them.

Next up: figuring out where to go. Our West Virginia Bureau of Public Health colleagues had recommended that we focus our assessments on the city of Clarksburg-Bridgeport and the more rural Gilmer County. Clarksburg-Bridgeport, with a population of twenty-eight thousand, was considered a large city by West Virginia's standards, and it was hoped that our findings there would give us an idea of how well the state's larger cities supported physical activity and healthy eating. Gilmer County had only seven thousand residents; it would give us an indication of how a small, rural county was faring.

While we finished our preparations in Atlanta, the West Virginia Bureau of Public Health staff called the local health departments in Clarksburg-Bridgeport and Gilmer County. Both departments gave the nod, but informed us that they would not be able to participate in the fieldwork—they were too busy with bioterrorism planning.

Bioterrorism? West Virginia had the highest rate of hypertension, the second-highest rate of diabetes, and the third-highest rate of obesity in the United States, but the local health departments had no capacity to join a three-week effort aimed at an investigation to address the situation? I was incredulous. While increasing numbers of people were dying from these debilitating and dangerous health conditions, local health departments were engaged in planning for bioterrorist activity with infectious disease agents that in all probability would never be used to target a small rural county.

This was frustrating, to be sure, but nothing unusual. With funding scarce, health department officials frequently "follow the money." If there's funding for bioterrorism preparedness, staff will be hired and put to work. In both the United States and Canada, funding for local health departments to address chronic disease is often nonexistent, except through limited grants. It's an imperfect system, given that finding and then applying for those grants is a labor-intensive process. As a result, many limited-capacity local health departments—which are all too often found in areas with the highest rates of NCDs and their related risk factors and conditions—are unable to put energy into getting the non-routine funding for fighting those NCDs. Instead, they spend their time creating or maintaining programs from the long-standing funding that is routinely provided to them only for the control of infectious diseases.

It would have been nice to have the help of the local health departments, but the lack of it wasn't going to stop us. We buckled down and prepared for our three weeks on the ground. In each locale, we chose a representative sample of schools, worksites, restaurants, grocery stores, convenience stores, and streets. We looked for tools used in previous studies to observe the offerings of foods and beverages in stores and restaurants. We looked for tools used to interview worksite and school staff. We used Google Maps to plot a one-quarter-mile radius around each school and the ten largest worksites. Those maps were then printed onto eight-by-eleven sheets of paper and placed on an ever-growing stack. Next came the painstaking work of numbering every street segment, the section of street between any two intersections. These hundreds of numbers would eventually correspond with the worksheet that at least two people in the field would complete for every segment, assessing and recording measures associated with walkability: sidewalk width and conditions, traffic speed limits, the number of cars speeding by, and land uses (what types of buildings sat on those streets and what services they offered).

Finally, we figured out our staffing needs. Since the EIS program generally supported a maximum of twenty-one days in the field for outbreak investigation teams, we needed to estimate how many people it would take to complete the work within that timeframe. We concluded that two to three team members from the CDC along with several people from the West Virginia Bureau of Public Health would do the trick. Andrea Sharma and I would be on site for the entire three weeks. Judd Fleisch, a medical student doing an elective with the CDC, was keen to accompany us for the first half of our trip, and Michele Maynard—a native of Gilmer County—would take over when Judd had to leave.

On our first morning in Charleston, Judd, Andrea, and I made our way to the West Virginia Bureau of Public Health. We were greeted in the lobby by Kerry Kennedy, director of the bureau's obesity program. She brought us upstairs to a conference room filled with twenty or so people, a combination of her staff and volunteers from other programs who were eager to head into the field with us. Some of Kerry's core staff would be with us almost daily over the next three weeks, while others would pitch in for one morning or afternoon. They would provide the additional help we needed, and, in turn, they would be trained in field data collection methods.

This was our only training day, and we had no time to waste. Not only did our volunteers need to learn how to use our data collection tools, but some of the tools themselves also needed final testing with field staff. On this first day, we learned that our restaurant audit form wasn't up to snuff. Our plan had been to look at the menus and use the form to capture information like the number of entrées on offer with one, two, or three servings of fruits and vegetables. That proved a nearly impossible task. Menus often don't accurately describe what's served in the main course, and rarely do they reveal how much of a side will be served. So, even if carrots are listed as a side, we could rarely tell if there would be a ¼ cup (half serving) or a ½ cup (full serving) of sliced carrots, or even just a garnish of one or two carrot sticks arranged on the plate. Andrea and I looked at each other and shook our heads. Why hadn't we thought of this? We'd run out of time in Atlanta before we'd had a chance to test this final tool. We'd just assumed it would work, since it had been used in a previous study. We'd never thought about the difficulties in garnering such quantified information from a menu.

We had to come up with a different form—and fast. Luckily, West Virginia's Bureau for Public Health had developed a menu assessment tool for a previous study. Kerry walked to her office, clicked through her computer files, and came back with the form in hand. We all sat down to review it, surrounded by the take-out menus we had gathered that day. We compared the form's list of items to record with the information available on the take-out menu of a pizza-and-pasta joint. Very quickly, we realized we needed to remove items such as "preparation methods" from the form. Were the potatoes that came with the chicken marsala deep-fried, pan-fried, roasted, or boiled? We couldn't always tell. We also decided to add a few questions for restaurant staff, to help suss out information that might not be available on the menu. For example, we'd found that although the restaurants we'd visited that afternoon all had milk on hand, it was rarely listed on the menu. But if you asked your server, they would happily tell you what types were available (whole, 2 percent, 1 percent, skim, chocolate!) and bring you a glass.

Our first day ended on a high note. We'd practiced, tested, and revised. Our staff and volunteers were ready to go, and we believed that our tools were now the best they could be for the tasks at hand. We headed back to the hotel, confident that we were ready.

Our first stop was Clarksburg-Bridgeport. After two hours of uneventful highway driving through hilly, green terrain, Andrea, Judd, and I arrived at the Holiday Inn that would be our home base for the next week and a half. At the time of our visit, Clarksburg-Bridgeport, in Harrison County, was a city of twenty-eight thousand residents. It had fifteen public schools and housed seven of the ten largest worksites in the county. Prior to the field visit, the West Virginia Bureau of Public Health team had contacted all fifteen schools: eight had agreed to a visit, five had refused, and two did not return their calls. The bureau had also contacted five additional Harrison County public schools, nearby but outside of Clarksburg-Bridgeport. They'd managed to reach only three of the seven large worksites, and two of those had agreed to participate. Both were private-sector worksites. One employed more than five hundred people, the other more than eighteen hundred. Appointment dates and times were set.

West Virginia is known for its many "hollows," and Clarksburg-Bridgeport is nestled in a large valley between rolling, tree-covered hills. The city was settled in the 1770s, and its long history is reflected in its gridded street pattern and old and narrow two- and three-story brick buildings in the downtown core. Where old buildings had been torn down, the streets had been widened and much larger and bulkier mid-rise concrete structures had been built. As we made our way to our two worksites, the small, pedestrian-friendly storefronts of downtown gave way to very large facilities. One of our sites was a nondescript multistory building, the other a sprawling single-story operation. Both housed frontline staff, support staff, and managers.

As tour guides showed us through the sites, we asked questions and made note of what we saw. In the multi-story facility, there was no encouragement for people to use the stairs (lack of even inexpensive signage is a common problem in North American buildings). Despite the size of the two employers—and their building sites, where space did not appear to be at a premium— no onsite exercise or shower facilities were available, and there were no policies to support employee fitness (although one worksite did subsidize employee gym memberships, an offer that studies show is generally taken up by only a small percentage of employees). Both sites fared better on nutrition supports, with lunchrooms and cafeterias providing salad offerings. One of the two also offered other vegetables, fresh fruit, and low-fat items in the cafeteria, and provided nutrition information.

Our school visits followed a similar pattern, though without the tour guide. Upon arrival, our team would typically head to the main office, where we'd interview the principal or assistant principal, as well as the physical education teacher and the food-services manager or personnel. We asked questions we thought would capture the healthiness of the foods served; specifically, we asked about the deep-frying of foods in the school kitchens.

Without fail, we were told that no deep-frying occurred. If we were visiting over the lunch hour, we'd then observe as food was served in the cafeteria, and this tended to be an eye-opening experience. When we saw the cafeteria items and menus, it became clear that the schools were routinely serving items such as chicken nuggets, french fries, and corn dogs. When we'd asked about the cooking methods, the staff had responded as though they were doing the cooking; in reality, the meals served were essentially pre-cooked food items, many battered and pre-fried, that the school food staff would then bake to heat up and serve.

We noticed that most of the schools had vending machines for students, and that none contained fruit or vegetables. The most commonly observed items were potato chips, cookies, cakes, and pastries. The beverage machines were no better. They usually featured colorful, branded advertising from the company that supplied the machine and were stocked with sugar-sweetened sodas and fruit drinks. Some also had fruit juice and water. We asked ourselves why children needed to buy water that could be provided out of a tap, especially since there were no drinking water safety issues in Clarksburg-Bridgeport. Fruit juice is no longer recommended for children by the American Academy of Pediatrics since it contains mostly sugar, though it's naturally occurring sugar, and sodas and fruit drinks are certainly not recommended. So why would schools provide such machines? We asked the principals. They confessed—some sadly, their ears flushing red with embarrassment—that the money from the vending machines was used to help fund field trips and extra-curricular activities. As it turned out, not only did the schools receive the machines for free, but they were also *paid* by the companies supplying them and advertising on them. Though well-intentioned, the fundraising efforts undertaken by these schools—including drives that routinely sold chocolate, candy, and cookies, but almost never fruits or vegetables—were putting children at risk. What chance did these kids have to make healthy choices?

Leaving the cafeteria, we'd make our way through locker-lined hallways to the gym. We'd ask the physical education teachers how much PE time their school offered. Thanks to our background research in Atlanta, we knew that West Virginia had recently passed legislation requiring elementary schools to provide at least thirty minutes of PE at least three days per week, while middle schools needed one full period per day for one semester each year (raising the question, "What about the other half of the school year?"), and high school students were required to take at least one full-credit course. While these requirements were woefully inadequate when compared to the recommendations of the National Association of State Boards of Education (NASBE)—which at the time called for 150 minutes or more per week of PE at elementary schools, and at least 225 minutes per week at middle and high schools—the majority of schools we visited still did not meet them. In fact, not a single elementary school we visited met the state requirements, and no high school met NASBE recommendations nor did they offer PE at all in the four years of study. We were certainly a long way from the U.S. Department of Health and Human Services guidelines that tell us children and youth should get at least sixty minutes of moderate-to vigorous-intensity physical activity every day in order to be healthy. It seemed that the schools in West Virginia—where the children spent most of their days—were not doing their part to support a physically active lifestyle.

When we pulled out our audit forms to document the physical activity facilities, we found that while the majority of schools had a gymnasium, some did not. Some had no outdoor play areas, though these were in the minority. On occasion, we were struck by how the paltry general PE programming at some schools contrasted with the state-of-the-art facilities geared toward the training and performance of their prized athletes. The take-away? If you were athletically inclined and exhibited a talent for sport, you'd be encouraged to get even fitter; if not, you'd get few supports to get and stay fit and would, in all likelihood, gain weight over time.

We also inquired about whether students could easily walk or bike to school. The vast majority of schools reported hazards for walking and bicycling, with the amount of traffic and traffic speed at the top of that list. A lack of bike trails was also a commonly identified issue, and in the more rural areas just outside of Clarksburg-Bridgeport we heard about an inadequate number of sidewalks. When schools actually had a walking or bicycling policy, these policies usually *prohibited* walking or cycling to school, owing to concerns about road safety.

Amid these depressing findings, our team took to the streets and sidewalks ourselves. We audited every street segment we had mapped out. Back in our planning stage, we'd chosen to focus on the quarter-mile radius around our sites, since previous studies had shown that most people were willing to walk to a destination if it was no more than five or ten minutes from their home or worksite. At regular adult walking speeds, five minutes usually corresponds to a quarter-mile, and ten minutes to a half-mile.

We assessed a total of 692 road segments in Clarksburg-Bridgeport. On sunny days, on cloudy days, on drizzly, gray days—dressed in our usual working attire of khakis or jeans, T-shirt layered with sweatshirt layered again with a wind-blocking, water-resistant shell, and an extra poncho in our backpacks just in case—our teams would head out to a school or worksite, even the ones that had refused an interview. There, we'd pull out the maps we had prepared with the numbered road segments. We'd walk the lowest-numbered segment first and then move up sequentially. We'd stop at a mid-block position that allowed us to observe most of the street between two intersections. Then, we'd start to record data. What types of buildings were around us? Was there housing close enough to a school to allow children to walk or bike? What about near the worksites? Was there a mix of housing types such as single-family homes and apartments? Buildings that house multiple families, like apartments or townhomes, increase the population density of a neighborhood, and population density, in turn, often increases the likelihood that services settle in and survive. Were there other offices and services in the area? Were there parks, playgrounds, recreation facilities? Banks and dry cleaners and post offices? What about grocery stores, convenience stores, and restaurants that kids in the school or adults in worksites could walk to? We found that 60 percent of the worksites we visited had restaurants within a five-minute walk. That was the good news. The bad news was that unhealthy food choices abounded: the majority of schools had convenience stores nearby, and a third had fast food restaurants within a five-minute walk. Of the worksites, 80 percent had convenience stores clustered around them, double the number that had grocery stores nearby.

We also recorded the conditions of the buildings. Were they boarded up or deserted, leading those who might walk by to feel unsafe? We checked for streetlights, which of course are vital for visibility and safety at night. We noted posted speed limits, and pulled out our clicker-counters to measure traffic volume. We'd check whether or not there was a sidewalk; if there was, we'd pull out our tape measures to record its width and make notes on its condition. Was it well-paved or cracked, clear for walking or full of obstructions, like posts and trees, that would pose barriers for people with walkers, wheelchairs, and strollers? We found that over one-third of the street segments around schools had no sidewalks, and even when sidewalks were present, about 40 percent had only poor or fair walkability. Things were even worse around the worksites, with nearly 90 percent of street segments lacking sidewalks.

Grocery and convenience stores were also on our list. We'd hit the produce section first, to count the varieties of fresh vegetables and fruits available. We recorded their appearance. Did they look fresh and enticing, or were they old and wilted? Next up were the meat aisles, to document whether the supermarket offered alternatives to higher-fat and red meat animal protein, like skinless chicken breasts, ground turkey, and fresh fish. We looked for whole wheat and high-fiber breads as alternatives to white bread. Finally, we headed to the dry goods shelves, on the hunt for items like whole wheat pasta as high-fiber choices. We used the same audit form at convenience stores, where we noted just how different the offerings were. For the most part, we found no vegetables, no fruit, no healthier options like high-fiber grains, but lots of chips, cookies, and soda.

Finally, we audited the area's restaurants. We'd ask for an eat-in menu and a take-out menu. Where the two were identical, we'd leave with the take-out menu and complete our audit forms in the car or back at the hotel. Where the menus were different, we would conduct the audit there. In fast food restaurants, we stood where we could see the menu board and filled out our forms, straining our necks to peer over the sometimes long lines of customers. Fast food restaurants comprised about half of the restaurants audited in Clarksburg-Bridgeport, with the other two major categories being "pizza" and "casual dining." We found that while many restaurants offered vegetables, not all did, and few offered fruit, healthy messages, or nutrition information. On the other hand, many offered "supersized" options.

Each evening, we returned to our hotel weary from walking. After dinner, Judd, Andrea, and I would convene in whatever room was serving as our "headquarters." We'd boot up our laptops, scoop up about a third of the day's completed forms, and start entering the data into the Excel spreadsheets and databases we'd created. It would be close to or after midnight when we'd finally say good night. Back in my own room, I'd fall asleep as soon as my head touched the pillow.

After a week and a half in Clarksburg-Bridgeport, we had completed our assessments. Our findings were telling. We'd learned that the majority of schools had not implemented the new state requirements for physical education, even though these standards were already well below national recommendations. We found that school cafeterias served many pre-fried frozen foods to their kids, and that on-site vending machines stocked with unhealthy choices and featuring paid advertisement of sugary drink products were used as fundraising vehicles. We found that many schools—and worksites—were surrounded by convenience stores and fast food restaurants that provided yet more exposure to unhealthy foods. We found that supermarkets—which did carry many varieties of healthy products like fruits and vegetables—were less available near schools and worksites than convenience stores, which carried none of these healthy foods. As for walking and bicycling for transportation, the schools that had policies on these items actually prohibited or discouraged these active transportation modes, citing hazards like traffic volumes and speeds, and inadequate sidewalks and bicycling trails. Worksite lunchrooms and cafeterias did provide salad offerings, but not necessarily other vegetables or fruits, or nutrition information. Supports for active living—even inexpensive signage to encourage stair use, or provision of onsite spaces for exercise within large work buildings—were also lacking.

After a week and a half of surveying Clarksburg-Bridgeport, we had to wonder: Would rural Gilmer Country tell us a different story?

Midway into our three-week adventure, we drove through the warm morning, a slight haze in the air. We cut through foothills and more hollows as we neared Gilmer County and Glenville, its main town. Though the scenery was beautiful, the poverty of some of the land's inhabitants was apparent.

We'd received permission to visit four of the ten largest worksites in the county. All were multi-story buildings. Three of the four had elevators. None encouraged people to use the stairs with signage (which all the evidence indicates is an effective intervention), but two provided shower facilities and three had both onsite indoor exercise facilities and fitness-oriented programs for their employees. All provided staff lunchrooms, and one had a cafeteria that reported offering salads, fruit, low-fat items, and nutrition information.

Four of the five schools in Gilmer County were elementary schools; the other was a combined middle and high school. We were impressed to find that none had a vending machine selling snacks, and only one had introduced a vending machine with beverages. Although none of the schools met NASBE recommendations for PE, all of the elementary schools met the recently passed state requirements. All had a gymnasium, and most had outdoor play spaces. All reported selling food (mostly chocolate and candy) to raise money. Unlike Clarksburg-Bridgeport, where fast food outlets and convenience stores surrounded schools, in Gilmer County none of the schools had food premises nearby—a good thing when it comes to avoiding exposure to unhealthy food.

We once again made our way into restaurants, grocery stores, and convenience stores. While nearly half of the restaurants in the county were "casual dining" spots as opposed to fast food outlets (an inversion of what we'd found in Clarksburg-Bridgeport), our other findings were similar. Salads and vegetables were available at the majority of restaurants we visited, but not all. Fruit was rarely available. Nutrition information was generally absent, and not a single restaurant we visited offered healthy-eating messages on their menus. In contrast, nearly half offered "supersized" options, usually for their unhealthiest items, like soda and french fries. In grocery stores, an average of more than twelve varieties of vegetables and fifteen varieties of fruit were counted—a result that matched what we'd found in Clarksburg-Bridgeport and also coincided with research associating grocery store access with healthier diets and lower body weights. Because the county had only two large grocery stores, convenience stores here were more likely to have some vegetables and fruits, although the average was only one variety of fruit and two varieties of vegetables.

Out on the streets, we recorded our observations of all 134 street segments within Glenville. We also assessed 16 other road segments in rural Gilmer County, chosen because they fell within a quarter-mile radius of a school or large worksite. We found ourselves walking hilly terrain, at once scenic and tiring. Houses were found within a five-minute walk of schools and large worksites. Stores were also found near all worksites, and the majority of worksites had good access to restaurants. Only one was situated close to a grocery store, but three had convenience stores in the vicinity. Despite the number of destinations within walking distance, there were few sidewalks. No street segment within a quarter mile of nine of the ten largest worksites in Gilmer County had a sidewalk, and more than 40 percent of those street segments were determined to be busy.

The situation on school-zone streets was similar. Despite having housing nearby, fewer than 10 percent of street segments surrounding schools had sidewalks. Of those streets without sidewalks, nearly 40 percent in Glenville and roughly 66 percent outside of Glenville were determined to be busy—a reality than runs counter to the idea that traffic in rural areas is quiet and slow. These streets were anything but. They would not have been safe for pedestrians to use without a sidewalk, and indeed, we saw few to no pedestrians on them. Every day, opportunities for children and adults to achieve physical activity through walking were being lost. And when healthy choices are not safe choices, they're not really choices at all.

On our third Sunday in West Virginia, as a break from work, Andrea, Michele, and I decided to go hiking at the Cedar Creek State Park. Brochures boasted of fourteen miles of hiking trails, just minutes from Glenville. It was a warm, sunny day, and the drive to the park took us through grassy, tree-lined, rolling hills. We parked in an almost empty lot and went in search of our trail. We found swimming pools, playgrounds, basketball courts, and baseball fields that were also largely empty, despite the beautiful weather. Here and there, a family picnicked around a barbecue pit, sending the smell of hamburgers and hot dogs wafting our way. Finally, we found signs indicating trails that began at a clearing and appeared to lead up into the hills. We picked one sign and began to follow the path behind it. Almost instantly, we were brought to a halt. The trail was overgrown with tall grass and dense trees. We chose another trailhead; again, within a few feet, we had to turn back. We tried a third trail. No luck. We gave up, walked back to our car, and returned to our hotel, disappointed. Our much-needed recreational exercise break was not going to happen.

Our three weeks in the field whizzed by. Before we knew it, our time in West Virginia had come to an end, and a mountain of work awaited us in Atlanta as we set about compiling our findings into a report.

On June 2, just a few weeks after we arrived home, CDC director Julie Gerberding announced our study at a press conference. The *New York Times* broke the story, stressing the unprecedented nature of our work: "For the first time," health reporter Gina Kolata wrote, "the Centers for Disease Control and Prevention has sent a team of specialists into a state, West Virginia, to study an outbreak of obesity in the same way it studies an outbreak of an infectious disease." In the days that followed, the story spread to CNN, the Associated Press, and countless other American media outlets; in the U.K., the *Guardian* picked it up. The Community Preventive Services Task Force asked to see our findings.

It would take months to analyze fully the data we'd collected, and to truly document why West Virginia was at the center of the obesity outbreak. But those of us who'd had "boots on the ground" already knew what to expect. Having visited schools, worksites, supermarkets, convenience stores, and restaurants, having walked the streets around these premises, having walked on Cedar Creek State Park's unusable, overgrown trails, we knew that our data would reflect just what we had experienced: that the healthy choices that people wanted to make and the healthy choices people wanted their children to have were not easily made. In West Virginia, the deck was stacked against those who wanted to live healthier lives. Was the same true of other cities in North America and around the world? Was this the *real* reason behind our current—and ever-worsening—obesity epidemic?

My time as a disease detective in West Virginia helped me to see clearly what I'd suspected for a long time: our cities and workplaces and schools were inherently unhealthy. In the same way that unsanitary conditions in eighteenth-century London led to outbreaks of infectious diseases like cholera, unhealthy living conditions in twentieth- and twenty-first-century cities around the world were leading to outbreaks of non-communicable diseases like obesity and its related conditions. We put a stop to many of those infectious-disease outbreaks through the use of public health programs and initiatives. Now, the time had come to take those lessons and apply them to the prevention of our deadly NCDs.

For more than a decade now, I have been trying to do my part. In public health departments and as a consultant, I have worked with communities and organizations to bring attention to the ways that our built environment—our buildings, streets, neighborhoods, and their amenities—can better enable healthy lifestyles. After years of working in my own silo, and not finding much support for my ideas, I now have allies around the world—men and women who, like me, believe that in order to tackle obesity and its related conditions, we need to change the conversation we have been having for the last fifty years. We must recognize that we are not alone in the battle to stay fit and healthy, and that solving the problem will require a concerted, cooperative effort across many disciplines. It will require government action, community action, and action on the part of individuals who feel strongly about creating a world where we all have the ability to make healthy choices. It will mean making fundamental changes to the ways we can eat, build, move, and play. This work is underway in many cities around the world, in myriad creative and inspiring ways, and I'm excited to share some of them with you here. System-wide changes don't come easily, or quickly. If we're truly going to change the conversation we've been having about our obesity problem, the key is to get as many people talking as possible. After all, there's strength in numbers.

PART ONE

HOW WE EAT

There's no denying the link between what we eat and what we weigh. At its most basic, obesity is the result of eating more than we can effectively burn off. In other words, the calories-in/calories-out equation is tilted in favor of calories-in. When that happens once in a while—a splurge here or there, a "treat"—it's likely no big deal. But when a "treat" like junk food becomes a regular occurrence—when we're overeating every day—over the course of months or years our weight creeps up. And once we get to the point where we're more than 20 percent over our ideal weight for our height . . . well, that's generally the point when we have tipped beyond being merely overweight to becoming obese.

How we eat, then, is clearly an important front in our battle against obesity. But it's not enough to simply make food the enemy. And it's certainly not enough to go merrily on our way, believing that willpower and dedication are our only weapons when it comes to managing our diets. Yes, weight gain can be the result of poor food choices, but what if the person choosing doesn't have the information he or she needs to make good choices? Or, worse, what if a poor choice is the only "choice" available?

If this is a fight we are truly going to win, we need to better arm ourselves. And we can start by ensuring three fundamentals when it comes to healthy living access, affordability, and information where and when we need it.

1 | CALORIE LABELING

KNOWLEDGE IS POWER

IN JUNE 2006, with the outbreak investigation in West Virginia complete, I sold my car, packed my bags, handed in my apartment keys, and boarded the subway for Atlanta's Hartsfield-Jackson International Airport. I was on my way to one of the key birthplaces of public health in the United States, New York City, where I'd accepted a position with the Department of Health and Mental Hygiene. Despite its antiquated name, the department had a growing reputation for taking on current-day public health problems. Not too long before my arrival, it had tackled a particularly thorny issue in an initiative hailed as a model for the world: smoking had been banned from all indoor spaces, including restaurants and bars.

I'd followed the department's work on this front with interest. The election of Michael Bloomberg as mayor in 2001 had brought with it the appointment of Dr. Thomas Frieden, a health commissioner who shared the mayor's dedication to data-driven decisions. And the data on smoking was clear: tobacco use was the leading cause of death among Americans. By 2002, when the new administration took office, the data also clearly showed that secondhand smoke was a health hazard, and that a smoking ban in indoor public spaces and workplaces was not only needed but also desired by both smokers and nonsmokers alike. Furthermore, the evidence suggested that smoking bans could also help the many smokers who wanted to quit.

Policies and programs were developed to prevent teens from starting to smoke, and to support those who wanted to quit to do so faster and more successfully. Nicotine replacement therapy, in the form of a gum or patch, was being shipped out, at no cost, to a great many members of the public who'd requested it during specified campaign periods. The city sales tax on cigarettes was also raised, and then raised again. These environmental and policy measures were coupled with hard-hitting media campaigns, and the result was a precipitous drop in smoking rates. Around the world, public health departments took note and began to wonder if they, too, could make a change. Before long, many other cities and countries were banning smoking in their indoor spaces.

I was inspired by the department's success. This was precisely the type of work that made the public health field so appealing to me. A problem had been identified and analyzed, and a broad-spectrum solution—involving interventions, outreach, and effective messaging—had been put into motion. The public health department's response to the threat posed by tobacco use was completely in tune with the work I'd just completed in West Virginia, and I was eager to collaborate with this forward-looking team that was obviously ready and able to tackle the toughest modern epidemics.

Target: Obesity

By the time I arrived in New York, the health department, having made gains against smoking, had turned its attention to obesity. As the second leading cause of death in the United States, obesity was clearly a crisis, and a worsening one at that.

Obesity is the result of unhealthy weight gain, and unhealthy weight gain is the result of an energy imbalance—that good old calories-in/calories-out equation. The number of calories we burn is determined in large part by the amount of physical activity in our daily lives. For the purposes of disease prevention, adults need to accumulate at least 150 minutes per week of moderate-intensity physical activity (cycling, brisk walking, etc.), or 75 minutes of vigorous-intensity activity (running or aerobics), and children need at least 60 minutes per day of moderate- to vigorous-intensity physical activity. But studies show that the majority of people do not meet these goals. In Canada, ParticipACTION estimates that only 15 percent of Canadian adults and 5 percent of Canadian children currently meet physical activity recommendations for health. And studies suggest that when the goal is not just disease prevention but weight control, the need for routine physical activity may be even greater, requiring in the order of 40 to 90 minutes per day in adults.

Unfortunately, we don't move nearly as much as we used to. Not so long ago, we farmed or fished or worked at manual labor without the help of machines. Our kids walked or biked to school, and spent countless hours playing outside. Under these conditions, caloric expenditures (calories-out) were high, and there was room for higher caloric consumption (calories-in). But things have changed. These days, many of us work at jobs that require sitting at a desk for long hours. The car is now the main mode of transportation in many cities, and even more so in suburbs and rural areas. Even farming and laboring jobs now often use machinery that people sit on for prolonged periods. And leisure time is often spent on the couch. Combined, these shifts in behavior have led to a drop in our daily caloric expenditures—just as our caloric consumption has increased with changing food marketing and retail trends and consumption habits. People are eating at restaurants more and more, and ever-larger portion sizes are being offered to—even forced upon—consumers.

No wonder we're in the grip of an obesity epidemic.

The problem, of course, is that efforts to help people combat obesity and weight gain have long proven unsuccessful. Health education for behavior and lifestyle change has had limited effectiveness. Though health education can increase awareness, study after study has shown that it is seldom able to produce and sustain changes in behavior on its own. People need practical help to undertake and maintain healthy behaviors.

The health department knew it had to provide more community environmental supports, to change the environment to make healthier behaviors easier to accomplish in daily life. The question, then, was twofold: What do we do, and how do we do it? Does it make sense to start with the environment for food, or for physical activity, or both? What foods and what premises should be targeted? These questions were not commonly being addressed by local health departments elsewhere—there were no clear role models to follow. So, New York City turned to the data and science that was available at the time.

Taking On the Take-Out

I arrived for my first day on the job on a beautiful July morning after the Independence Day celebrations. I had been assigned a new, oddly shaped office on the fourteenth floor of a mid-rise, City-owned building at the corner of Lafayette and Duane Streets in downtown New York. The building had recently been renovated to accommodate the growing number of staff being hired by the Bureau of Chronic Disease Prevention and Control. From my small window, I could see sunlight shimmering off the glass of the many buildings surrounding me, and the streets of Lower Manhattan below.

My very first meeting was later that morning in the third-floor boardroom of a neighboring building at 125 Worth Street. This 1800s structure, with a beautiful old exterior and a drab, out-dated interior, had headquartered the city's health department from its start. As the boardroom filled with assistant commis-sioners and their directors, the Health commissioner, Dr. Frieden, flanked by his staff, began his review of the work of the last three months. On the table in front of him was a large black binder filled with summaries of the many initiatives he was to be updated on, every page of which he had read. One assistant commissioner after another rattled off updates, turning to their directors for details when the commissioner questioned them further. It appeared I had arrived in the midst of some frantic work on new food initiatives. Among them were attempts to craft new regula-tions on calories.

In some ways, we were starting from a position of strength. Health education had made people aware of the connection between calories and weight gain, and consumers were now used to checking the labels on processed and packaged foods for calo-rie information. But what about other foods? Would it be possible to provide calorie information for non-packaged foods?

It sounded like a great idea, but it certainly wasn't straight-forward. The biggest challenge here was determining where we could intervene.

Many public health departments, including New York City's, have the authority to carry out inspections in restaurants and day-cares, and are responsible for licensing and regulating these premises. They have the power to enforce a reasonable standard of food-safety practices in public eating establishments, and safety and hygiene standards in daycares. By and large, these rights had been given to governments because people accept these forms of government interference in exchange for the guarantee that their health will be safeguarded against food-borne illness, and their children's health against safety and infection control violations.

Restaurants, then, were a logical starting place: one of the department's first projects would be to get calorie information to the public for restaurant food.

Research suggested the effort would be worth it. People tend to underestimate the calories found in restaurant meals (I've certainly been guilty of this myself!). On days when adults and children eat fast food, they consume, on average, over 150 calories more than on other days. When we eat meals prepared outside the home, we have less (and sometimes no) control over the type and quantity of ingredients used, how they are cooked, and how much we are served. To make food tasty, restaurants often add more of the salt, fats, sugars, and other ingredients we use sparingly at home. When going out to restaurants was an occasional treat, this underestimation probably wasn't doing much harm, but these days, we eat many meals outside the home. Fast food sales have grown particularly quickly: in 1970, the fast food industry was worth $6 billion; by 2000, that figure had grown to $110 billion.

Fortunately for a science-driven health department, at the same time that the fast food industry was growing—along with obesity in both adults and children—research was being done on effective interventions for behavior change. Faced with the rise of non-communicable diseases and the need to identify evidence-based public health interventions for whole populations that could be carried out in community settings outside of health care services, the U.S. Department of Health and Human Services created a new task force in 1996, modeled after the U.S. Preventive Services Task Force. The Preventive Services Task Force had been charged with reviewing evidence-based interventions for preventive services and procedures in clinical or health care settings—interventions such as Pap smears every three years for women between the ages of twenty-one and sixty-five, and screening for high blood pressure in adults aged eighteen years and over. The new Community Preventive Services Task Force was similarly charged with reviewing the scientific evidence to identify and recommend community-level interventions that could be conducted to affect outcomes in whole populations.

By 2001, the task force had released a list of recommendations for physical activity based on sufficient or strong levels of scientific evidence. Among these was a whole category of interventions called "environmental and policy change approaches." And among the environmental approaches recommended for physical activity were interventions that provide "point-of-decision information." The review showed that, for physical activity, when information encouraging active options like stair use is posted at points where people make decisions about behaviors—near elevators, escalators, and stairs—people increase their physical activity. Across many studies, stair use, for example, has been shown to increase by 50 percent when information is present. In 2004, a review article showed that among the environmental factors that appeared to change consumer behaviors related to healthy eating, those with the strongest evidence of effectiveness included access to healthy food and posted point-of-decision information. So, making health information available at decision points appeared to be supported not only for increasing awareness but also for actual behavior change. Reminders help people with the choices they want to make for their health but which they might forget day to day in the course of their busy lives.

Making health information about food and food products available was not a new concept in 2006. In 1989, the U.S. federal government had passed the Nutrition Labeling and Education Act to improve the labeling of packaged foods. It was a great move for consumers, who could now make better-informed choices about the foods they were purchasing, but it also had an interesting side effect—one that we were very much aware of as we contemplated our own initiatives. Studies done following the implementation of the new labeling requirements showed that quantities of some less healthful ingredients in packaged foods, such as sodium and fat, decreased.

This was music to our ears—proof that the intervention we were considering, while benefiting consumers in the short term, might also create industry-wide changes that would support healthier living over the long term. Even with this evidence in hand, however, we weren't quite ready to make our move. Department and City lawyers had warned us that any attempt to mandate the clear posting of calorie information in restaurants would likely be met with opposition. In general, industry is sensitive to increased regulation, fearing a slippery slope, and will look for reasons to oppose it. In order to ensure that our efforts to intervene on behalf of consumers were successful, we needed as much evidence as possible to support our plan. Most importantly, we needed local evidence to supplement the studies based on research elsewhere.

And so the field studies began. Armed with university interns supervised by department staff, the health department got to work. With transit passes as their weapon of choice, the interns and staff swarmed onto subways and then dispersed into fast food restaurants. When customers completed their purchases, they would be approached and asked about their willingness to take a survey in exchange for a MetroCard offering a free subway ride. Some walked away, claiming they had no time. Some appeared annoyed at having been bothered. But others agreed. The survey was short—just one question asking if the participants had seen calorie information at the restaurant they'd just left. Customers were also asked if they were willing to part with their meal purchase receipts.

The surveys done before the introduction of regulatory changes in New York City found that fewer than 4 percent of fast food restaurant customers were getting calorie information, despite claims from the industry that this information was available. McDonald's, for example, proudly stated that it listed calorie information on a web page that got two thousand hits per day . . . which translates to 0.004 percent of its fifty million customers a day! There was one exception, however: 32 percent of Subway's customers did report seeing calorie information. Why such a big difference? When the restaurants were assessed, only Subway was providing calorie information in its restaurants on its menus and menu boards.

It's not as if the other chains were lying; they had tested their foods and beverages for nutrition content, including calories, and they were providing that information in various forms—on their website, in brochures, on the bottom of their tray-liners. But the study in New York also demonstrated that consumers were not receiving the information (who looks under tray-liners?). At Subway, however, where the information was prominently displayed with the menu, a significant number of customers were taking it in. The message was clear: information posted on menus had a much higher likelihood of reaching the consumer.

This wasn't the only innovative local study we used to justify our regulatory approach. Through the annual Community Health Survey, we had also begun collecting data on the health of the New York City population across its five boroughs. Using a process developed by and surveys adapted from the CDC, numbers from telephone directories were randomly chosen and dialed, and willing adults were asked to answer questions anonymously about demographic factors as well as various health markers, including weight and height, physical activity levels, dietary behavior, and other conditions like diabetes and high blood pressure. Measures of weight, height, and physical fitness in children were also added through data collected in physical education classes at schools. Supplementing all of this was data from hospitals and health care providers on diabetes. Diabetes A1C results, a blood test measure of whether people had diabetes and how well people were controlling their diabetes, had been made reportable by laboratories which processed such tests—just like serious infectious diseases such as cholera and tuberculosis—to the health department in New York City in December 2005. All of this data told the city's story: diabetes rates were high, and obesity rates were high in both adults and children—approximately 60 percent of adults and 40 percent of children were overweight or obese—and continuing to rise. In fact, in 2006, obesity and diabetes were the two health conditions worsening in New York City. These alarming figures underlined the need for population-level interventions and provided justification for the approach we were proposing.

With international, national, and now local studies in hand, our team sat down to craft a feasible regulation. Around the meeting table in the assistant commissioner's office, the small group working on this issue (four or five out of the staff of approximately one hundred people in the Bureau of Chronic Disease Prevention and Control) brainstormed: Which restaurants could be targeted? Which would need to be excluded? Where would the information be posted? What would the impacts be? After a lot of back and forth, we were finally ready, and in 2006, New York City made its move to become the first jurisdiction in the world to pass a calorie-labeling requirement for meals served in restaurants. Restaurants that already provided calorie information in some format—via website, brochure, on the back of the tray-liner, and so on—would be required by the proposed regulation to also post that information on menus and menu boards, next to and in the same size font as the price. We knew the regulation was an important start, but it was far from ideal. Many restaurants—including those that didn't already provide calorie information—would not be required to participate. Small mom-and-pop operations and restaurants with ever-changing menus, which could not afford to test their foods and beverages for nutrition information, were also not required to post it. Still, we had taken the first step, and we were proud of the work that had gone into getting to this stage.

As expected, it didn't take long for the restaurants to fight back. In 2007, the regulation was challenged by the New York State Restaurant Association. When court day arrived, the restaurant association lawyer, dressed in an impeccable, well-pressed suit, presented his clients' case. First, he argued, the City of New York had no jurisdiction to do this: food labeling was a federal concern. Not only that, but the City was violating the freedom of speech of his clients, the restaurant corporations, by preventing them from writing their menus as they wanted, with the information they wished to include. Then the middle-aged health department lawyer stood up. Despite his rumpled suit, he was articulate and well prepared. He presented the department's defense: the fast-growing obesity epidemic; the underestimation and over-consumption of calories in restaurants; the need to provide consumers with information so they could make informed choices; and on and on. My colleagues and I sat tensely in the courtroom.

The judge listened. He deliberated. And finally, he delivered his verdict: he struck down the regulation.

It was quite a blow. We were deflated—and exhausted. I remember feeling beaten. I remember wondering if all of our efforts would amount to nothing. Would the big corporations always win, because they had the biggest budgets for lawyers, the biggest budgets for advertising their products?

But we didn't give up. With a good night's sleep under our belts, we regrouped. Though the judge had struck down the regulation, he'd firmly stated that he did not agree with the restaurant association's arguments. Instead, the basis for his decision had been his concern that it unfairly singled out restaurants that already voluntarily provided calorie information. He explicitly affirmed the legal jurisdiction of the New York City health department to undertake a regulatory measure such as this, but he suggested that the regulation needed to be "restructured."

Fortunately for New York City, public health workers in the rest of the country—and even around the world—had been watching our work closely. In fact, some had already begun regulatory or legislative processes modeled after New York's. Just as our regulation was being struck down, Washington State's Seattle–King County passed its own regulation for required calorie labeling, targeting not restaurants that already provided this information voluntarily but one specific category: chains.

Chain Reaction

In many North American cities, chain restaurants dominate the dining-out landscape; in New York City, however, chains make up only 10 percent of restaurants. Despite this relatively low figure, they accounted for more than a third of the total restaurant traffic across the city's five boroughs, a larger share of visits than any other category. And many of the chain restaurants were fast food restaurants.

Where we eat matters. It determines what, how much, and even how quickly we eat. Do we have time to sit? Is it pleasant to do so? These considerations affect the speed at which we eat, and that speed can, in turn, affect how satisfied we feel. It takes time for the food we eat to be digested and for the sugars to be released into our bloodstream, stimulating the "satiety centers" in our brain. Eating slowly can help allow us to experience feelings of "fullness" before we overeat. With that in mind, the argument can be made that fast food restaurants, with their emphasis on speed and an "in and out" dining experience (some don't even have tables), may encourage overeating, creating an environment that prioritizes profits from turnover over health. In these settings, being informed about calorie counts is especially important. Having that information readily available as we grab a quick lunch between meetings could be the difference between consuming a 350-calorie grilled chicken sandwich or a 1,000-calorie burger, or between "supersizing" a much-craved serving of fries or settling for the small.

In the years leading up to the calorie-labeling regulations in the United States, chain restaurants had been busy trying to protect themselves from liability for their high-calorie, high-fat food products. In July 2002, a fifty-six-year-old man from the Bronx, New York, was the first to launch a broad-based lawsuit against the fast food chains for his poor health. He had developed diabetes and suffered a heart attack (his second), he claimed, after eating their food four to five times a week, not knowing the hazards these foods would pose. In particular, the suit stated, the restaurant chains had been negligent in not properly disclosing the ingredients that, consumed frequently, would lead to his health conditions. In November 2002, two teenagers sued McDonald's and the two franchises they frequently visited in the Bronx for their obesity, citing insufficient provision of necessary nutrition information as the basis for their legal action.

Though the obesity lawsuits were dismissed by the courts, the reaction they created in the industry presented opportunities for new strategies to be developed. In an effort to protect itself from possible liability, the industry began to test its food products and to make nutrition information available to its consumers (in the less-than-obvious ways we've discussed). And the availability of that information made calorie-labeling laws like the one passed in Washington State both feasible and affordable.

Encouraged by Seattle's success and by the judge's affirmation of jurisdiction and powers, we went back to work. We reviewed the judge's comments regarding how to redraft the regulation. We reviewed the wording of Seattle's new policy. We worked hard and quickly, and we soon had a new regulation to present.

In January 2008, for the second time, a regulation mandating calorie posting in restaurants was passed in New York City. This time, however, the policy was applied to restaurants with fifteen or more locations in the United States. Their outlets within the jurisdiction of New York City—Manhattan, the Bronx, Brooklyn, Queens, and Staten Island—now had to post calorie information on menus and menu boards, next to and in the same font size as the price. The New York State Restaurant Association once again launched a court action to oppose the new regulation, but this time, despite their claims of lack of feasibility ("there's not enough space on the menu or menu board for such information") or cost ("it would cost too much to change our menu or menu boards for just the New York City market"), restaurant opposition was struck down by the courts and the new regulations were upheld.

New York's victory seemed to embolden other jurisdictions. Since 2008, progress on calorie posting has accelerated across the United States. In 2010, Philadelphia passed similar legislation. In 2011, California enacted a state law for calorie labeling in restaurants. And in 2010, at the federal level, the U.S. Affordable Care Act's prevention package mandated the posting of calories and other potential nutrition information by chain restaurants with twenty or more outlets within the United States. That federal legislation also covers vending machine operators with twenty or more operational machines. On November 25, 2014, calorie-labeling regulations were released by the U.S. Food and Drug Administration covering not only fast food and sit-down chain restaurants and vending machines, but also supermarkets, convenience stores, and movie theaters. Widespread implementation and enforcement of the regulations across the U.S., however, did not occur until May, 2018, eight years after the law was passed. And other countries, like Canada, still need to follow suit.

Lessons Learned

The story of the calorie-labeling regulation process in chain restaurants in New York City provides several lessons for public health policy and the processes of environmental change.

One lesson is how this type of process can quickly turn into a cat-and-mouse game that, although frustrating, can open doors to change. The chain reaction caused by the restaurant industry's response to those obesity lawsuits—for example, making nutrition information publicly available—gave public health departments the leverage they needed to successfully intervene on behalf of consumers to be able to get the information where and when they need it most. Those of us who work in the field of public health can take comfort in the fact that being down doesn't necessarily mean being out.

A second lesson comes in the form of an old adage: If at first you don't succeed, try, try again. It took New York City several years, countless studies, untold hours of research and evaluation, and multiple trips to court to get the job done. But we did it. Apparently, tenacity—not to mention a healthy dose of stubbornness—is a necessary skill in public health.

And lesson number three? We had to wait a bit before learning that one, because there was still work to be done. Like any data-driven entity, like any entity devoted to the rigors of science, and like any entity accountable for the impacts of its actions, the New York City health department had to conduct evaluations. Yes, the evidence suggested that point-of-decision information could change behavior, that federal packaged-food-labeling rules had changed industry practices, and that calories displayed on menus and menu boards increased exposure to the information, but the question of whether the City's regulation had made a difference remained to be answered.

And so began the impact studies. Indeed, one could argue that they had begun even before the regulation itself had passed. Remember those meal purchase receipts the "army of interns" collected during the surveys done in preparation for the regulatory process? Well, when that army returned from their field visits with backpacks full of receipts and surveys, the health department evaluator got to work. Calories were calculated. Each receipt was matched to a survey question regarding how many individual meals had been purchased, and that information, in turn, was used to calculate the number of calories per meal. Before the regulation was even enacted, the department's evaluator had tabulated the average calories per meal. Across all restaurants, the result showed an average of 827 calories, with hamburger and fried chicken chains usually coming in at above 1,000 calories per meal.

Now, with the regulation firmly in place, we once again hired an enthusiastic group of student interns. After-regulation surveys were conducted with willing fast food customers, meal receipts were again collected, and the evaluator again calculated the average calories per meal, this time for purchases made *after* the passage and implementation of the regulation.

Although real-world studies are often imperfect since they occur outside of controlled environments such as laboratories, they are nevertheless important. Quite a number of studies have now been conducted on New York's and Seattle's calorie-labeling regulations, including those by researchers from universities in New York and elsewhere. In addition, voluntary calorie-posting initiatives have occurred in several settings, such as hospital and university cafeterias, and have been paired with research.

A review of the available studies in 2013 sums up the findings. First, consumers want this information. When surveyed, 76 percent of U.S. adults and 84 percent of New York City residents (after passage of the regulation) considered the information to be helpful. Yet when such information is not posted on menus and menu boards, few people see it. Backing up the research we'd accessed during the lead-up to the regulation, one study of eight restaurants with nutrition information available on site (on pamphlets, for example) but not on menus or menu boards indicated that less than 1 percent of patrons looked at the information. But where calorie information was posted on menus and menu boards—as it was in New York City and Seattle after the regulatory changes—the majority of customers in food chains (54 percent to 87 percent, in different studies) reported seeing the information. Furthermore, customers who reported using the information purchased fewer calories after the information was made available. It's worth noting, however, that the impact of calorie labeling may not be the same in all situations. Women, for example, appear to be more receptive than men to the information overall. And the outcome could differ depending on the type of food items purchased (the good news is that higher-calorie items may be most affected) and the type of chain restaurant (accounting for differences in the types of foods or beverages served). Available evidence does suggest, though, that the restaurant industry need not be too worried about the impacts on its bottom line: the regulation does not reduce restaurant revenue.

One key outcome of interest post-regulation was change to the restaurant food environment itself. I experienced this myself soon after the calorie-labeling law in New York was enacted. Stepping into a Starbucks one afternoon, I was pleased to see that I could now easily determine the number of calories in my latte, and debate, fully aware of the caloric consequences, whether a chocolate-chunk cookie was worth the splurge. But above and beyond that, I saw more of what we had hoped the legislation would help to accomplish: a change in food industry practices that would lead to the provision and promotion of more lower-calorie options.

As I stood in line looking at the menu, now with calories next to the prices, my eyes were drawn to a special "Skinny Menu" of lower-calorie items. I could opt for a skinny latte, a skinny cappuccino—you name it; there appeared to be a previously unavailable skinny version of almost every drink displayed prominently on the menu. What's more, Starbucks was actually *promoting* the lower-calorie items. In press releases after the regulation passed, the company announced that it had switched from whole milk to 2 percent as its default. Other restaurant chains also changed their ingredients; at Cosi, a switch from regular to low-fat mayonnaise saved up to 350 calories on some sandwiches. McDonald's too made changes, reformulating its large serving of french fries to drop the calorie count below 500. The industry, previously a challenger to the law, had now come on side—because it had to.

This, then, is the third lesson for public health policy: sometimes the law has to lead and industry will follow—even when it comes to providing customers with the choices that they want.

2 | FOOD DESERTS

THE IMPORTANCE OF ACCESS AND AFFORDABILITY

HAVING GOOD INFORMATION about the food you intend to consume is certainly important when it comes to battling obesity and its health consequences, but there are more basic issues that need to be addressed if we're truly going to win this war. In his best-selling book *The Omnivore's Dilemma*, Michael Pollan provides a succinct recipe for individual and societal health: "Eat food. Mostly plants. Not too much." But what if real food is lacking? What if plants aren't there for us to pick from our gardens or buy from our stores? What if everything that *is* there has too much salt, sugar, and fat, and will kill you if eaten regularly? Without access to healthy food choices—not to mention *affordable* healthy food choices—we are bound to fail.

Maria is a widowed single mom who lives with her three children in a one-bedroom apartment in the South Bronx. To make ends meet, she has been working two jobs for several years now—one at a McDonald's a few subway stops away, the other at a Burger King just down the street from her apartment. Yet she is barely making it. She wishes there were a supermarket nearby so she could buy her children proper food, but the nearest one is several miles away, too far for her to walk, and not located near a subway station. She has tried to go there before but found she had trouble lugging home the heavy bags, especially because the store is a twenty-minute walk from the nearest bus stop. Once a month or so she manages to carpool with a friend and does a bigger shop, but in the weeks in between she relies on neighborhood stores. She often visits the corner bodega for milk and white bread, for peanut butter and jelly, and for the boxed macaroni with the bright orange cheese powder that the kids love. She wishes the bodega would carry some fruits and vegetables, but it doesn't. She's aware that whole grain bread would be better for the kids, but the store doesn't carry that either. Sometimes she'll bring home the leftover burgers or chicken nuggets her employers are ready to throw out. She knows eating this way isn't healthy for the kids, or her. Her weight has been steadily creeping up, and she's made more than one New Year's resolution to try to eat better and to exercise. But, with the kids and her two jobs, she never seems to find the time. There are no gyms nearby, and the park they could walk to doesn't seem safe. Recently, on her way home from the subway on a Saturday morning in June, she noticed canopied stalls set up at the edge of the park. She wandered over to have a look and was thrilled to see fresh fruits and vegetables. But one look at the prices left her feeling crestfallen.

Maria is fictional, but her circumstances certainly aren't. Like many people in North America's biggest cities, inner cities and even suburban neighborhoods, Maria lives in a "food desert." The U.S. Department of Agriculture defines a food desert as a place where at least five hundred people, and/or at least 33 percent of the population, live more than a mile (equivalent to a twenty-minute walk with heavy bags) from the nearest grocery store or supermarket, thereby limiting the availability of fresh fruits, vegetables, and other whole foods. (In rural areas, the distance is set at more than ten miles.) It's estimated that

23.5 million people in the United States live in food deserts; of these, 13.5 million, like Maria, are considered low-income.

This lack of access to healthy food choices is bad enough on its own, but the situation is compounded by a related issue: an abundance of unhealthy choices. Newspaper stands now sell chips, cookies, and soda. Gas stations do too, often along with burgers, hot dogs, french fries, fried chicken, and pizza. Vending machines in many workplaces, even our hospitals, ensure that we are never safe from the onslaught of unhealthy foods and beverages. And, of course, fast food outlets are everywhere—there were more than 200,000 in the United States in 2018, and 27,000 in Canada (or more than ten per 10,000 population). In the United States, it's estimated that there are five fast food outlets for every one supermarket. Increasingly, we cannot avoid high-calorie, low-nutrient foods; these poor choices crowd out the few good choices that might exist, creating an unhealthy "food swamp" amid the food desert. And, like the food deserts they are so often found in, food swamps occur in particularly high concentrations in our poorest neighborhoods.

So why can't we just ignore all of that unhealthy stuff? Easier said than done, as it turns out. The science of nutrition is increasingly revealing how people respond to fat, sugar, and salt—common ingredients in all those highly processed and fast food choices that are so prevalent in food deserts and swamps. In *Salt, Sugar, Fat: How the Food Giants Hooked Us*, author Michael Moss interviews experts both working for and fighting against the food industry, who repeatedly tell us about "mouthfeel," the sensation of pleasure that food can produce through the right combination of these three ingredients. When these foods are readily available—and especially when they are cheap—it's a combination that most of us can't resist. And after we give in and indulge? Well, that's when we're plagued with guilt over what we feel is a moral failure, and we end up blaming ourselves for what we perceive as a lack of self-control.

And that's not even all of the bad news. Brian Wansink is a professor at Cornell University. I first heard Brian lecture at the Active Living Research conference in San Diego in 2003. In a breakout session, Brian told us about his research, conducted in a lab, showing that people are programmed to eat when food is available. "Even stale popcorn, and even when people say they aren't hungry," Brian told the small gathering. "As long as I supplied the food, people ate it." Talk about having the deck stacked against you! On the one hand, we've got fast food giants and food processors working hard to improve the tempting mouthfeel of their unreal foods; on the other hand, we've got our own biological imperative to eat.

Dr. Kim Morland, a researcher at New York's Mount Sinai Hospital, has studied food in this modern-day context. And her findings underline the repercussions of food deserts and swamps: in neighborhoods with supermarkets nearby, we find lower levels of obesity than in neighborhoods with lots of fast food outlets. Other researchers, too, have shown this in their studies. No wonder we're battling the bulge. Increasingly, though, we are not alone in the fight. Some of our cities have begun to push back against our inability to find places where real foods like fruits and vegetables can be bought or grown. And they're doing it with some tried-and-true weapons: creative thinking, cooperation, zoning, and money.

Building a Better Bodega

Candace Young and Sabrina Baronberg had been working together for a year or two when I arrived in New York in 2006. Candace, director of the city health department's Physical Activity and Nutrition Program, tag-teamed with her deputy director, Sabrina, to devise a number of initiatives to increase food choices for residents of the Big Apple. Studies undertaken by the health department in the South Bronx, in parts of Harlem, and in Brooklyn, particularly in their poorest neighborhoods, had revealed that these locations had the highest rates of obesity and diabetes in the city. Furthermore, supermarkets were lacking in many of the high-poverty neighborhoods, although bodegas and convenience stores abounded, selling cigarettes, alcohol, potato chips, cookies, and sodas. Since these bodegas were the neighborhood's predominant food stores, they also frequently carried items that residents might need to pick up in between journeys to a supermarket farther afield—things like bread and milk. The health department studies showed that while super-markets carried many varieties of vegetables, fruits, and whole-grain breads and pastas, bodegas usually did not. This finding lent credence to a link that was being explored in research like that conducted by Kim Morland: people who lived near super-markets had lower obesity rates and better diets than those who did not.

New York clearly had a food desert problem, and that problem was, in turn, contributing to issues with obesity and its conse-quences. The health department decided it needed to do some-thing concrete to help, something more than preach to people about eating better—it needed to make sure people could actu-ally heed that advice. After some more research and a bunch of brainstorming, the department came up with a multi-pronged approach. First, we would attempt to improve the offerings in bodegas and corner stores, thereby making healthier food and beverage choices available in neighborhoods without easy access to a supermarket. Second, we would work to make healthy choices available to even our lowest-income residents. And third, we would tackle the thorny issues of supermarket availability. The first item could potentially be achieved by reaching out to and working with bodega operators and other local businesses. The second and third would be more difficult, and would likely take longer. They would entail working not only with supermarket owners and operators, but also with departments outside health, such as the Mayor's Office, the Human Resources Administration, Economic Development, and City Planning. Candace and Sabrina opted to start with the first, most feasible initiative.

Sabrina was given the lead on the healthy bodegas project. She and her revolving team of interns—primarily students working toward a master's degree in Public Health at nearby universities like Columbia or NYU—began their outreach to bodega owners. Their first goal was the creation of educational and promotional materials that the owners could post in their stores to identify and promote healthier items. They found funding from the city to subsidize the costs to the bodega owners of some of the healthier food options, hoping this would encourage them to try stocking them and selling them at a relatively low price. Some bodega owners signed on to give the initiative a try; they posted the in-store information and promoted the healthy choices. As customers read the signs and bought the promoted and lower-priced items (chalk one up for point-of-decision prompting!), bodega owners realized that there was a genuine demand for these healthier items after all—now they had a strong incentive to continue stocking them. Once again, a broad-based approach involving education, government action, and community participation had worked.

The healthy bodega initiative has come a long way. Today, it is called Shop Healthy NYC! The Physical Activity and Nutrition Program—which split into the Active Living Program and the Nutrition Program—became the new Center for Health Equity. Shop Healthy NYC! now has two main components: training for stores willing to modify their inventory, placement, and promotion of healthier food options, and training for community groups and organizations to support bodega owners to offer healthier options. Community advocacy groups and organizations are encouraged to "adopt" a bodega and to use their influence with community residents to increase demand for and purchasing of healthier options at that location.

Health Bucks

The Shop Healthy NYC! initiative is clearly a success story, but on its own it's not enough. Access to healthier choices is one thing, but being able to afford them is another matter altogether. Calorie for calorie, fruits and vegetables are much more expensive today than low-nutrient, high-calorie processed food sold in prepackaged or fast food form. Studies of healthy food baskets in North America have shown that the foods that make up a healthy diet are not affordable for those living in poverty. And for many people in North America, living in poverty is a reality.

In Canada, nearly 5 million people live in poverty, with over 1.3 million children (1 in 5) impacted; in the United States, over 40 million people live in poverty. Statistics Canada has recently introduced the Market Basket Measure, or MBM, which establishes a threshold for low income based on the cost of a basket of goods and services needed to meet basic needs and achieve a modest standard of living.

In both the United States and Canada, the problem of not being able to afford food, let alone healthy food, has been growing over the last several decades. Modeled after similar initiatives in the United States, the first food bank in Canada opened in Edmonton in 1981. Though this was intended as a temporary solution to the issue of hunger and food insecurity that had started to creep into Canadian cities, more and more food banks have opened year after year, and they have become a permanent fixture in many Canadian cities. Decades of stagnant minimum wages have exacerbated the problem. In 1970s Canada, working roughly forty hours a week at a minimum-wage job would produce an income adequate to support the worker and one other person (e.g., a child) at Statistics Canada's poverty threshold; by the 1990s, minimum wage had fallen far behind inflation, and a person working at minimum wage needed to work over seventy hours a week to stay above the poverty line. Compounding this issue is the fact that many minimum-wage jobs are part-time jobs, so that workers need to cobble together two or three jobs just to make ends meet.

Sabrina and her colleagues were well aware of the statistics concerning poverty, and they were just as determined to tackle affordability as they were to tackle access. In 2005, the Physical Activity and Nutrition Program came up with a pretty creative solution to the problem: they decided to print their own money. The idea was to give these "Health Bucks" to partner organizations which, in turn, would make sure the "money" got into the hands of the many families living below the poverty line.

Knowing that access to supermarkets was an issue for many in high-needs neighborhoods, Sabrina and her team also worked to have the currency accepted by vendors at farmers' markets. The Health Bucks were each worth two dollars that would be added to a purchase of five dollars or more worth of fruits and vegetables. The farmers could then return the coupons to city administration and redeem two dollars for each one.

Easy, right?

No. It wasn't enough just to get the farmers to cooperate. Before Sabrina and her team even approached the farmers' market vendors about the Health Bucks program, the health department had to lay the groundwork. This involved working with New York City's newly hired Food Policy Coordinator (FPC). The FPC position had been created by the Mayor's Office in 2007 to ensure that policies needed to promote access to healthy food—policies that extended beyond the capability of any one department— would be coordinated. It seemed to be working; through such coordination, for example, the FPC was successfully creating more farmers' markets across the city, including expansions into New York's poorest neighborhoods.

This was music to Sabrina's ears—but now the trick was making sure that those markets could actually process food stamps and also accept the Health Bucks. The government department in New York City responsible for food stamps is the Human Resources Administration. The FPC encouraged them to provide the farmers with food-stamp processing machines and teach the farmers how to use them.

So, not exactly easy. But where there's a will, there's a way. In 2012, seven years after the launch of the Health Bucks program, 125 farmers' markets across the five boroughs of New York City were accepting food stamps. And all of them were accepting Health Bucks, too. Between 2005 and 2012, more than $1 million in Health Bucks were redeemed. By 2015, that number had more than doubled. That's $2 million spent not on fast or processed food but on healthier choices that might previously have been unaffordable.

Getting FRESH

The Health Bucks initiative is a perfect example of how much can be achieved through cooperation; when willing parties work together, so much good can be done. In 2008, as I began the difficult work of tackling the third prong in the City's approach to increasing access and affordability, I knew I was going to need buckets of cooperation in order to succeed.

The goal of the Food Retail Expansion to Support Health (FRESH) was to provide the much-needed sustenance of real and fresh food by either creating new supermarkets or expanding existing stores in the city's food deserts. The idea was to use tools that the city already had—particularly zoning and money—to get the job done.

Zoning is the regulatory planning tool that cities use to guide the form, land use, and availability of amenities in different neighborhoods. Zoning laws determine what types of buildings can be built within particular areas of a city, and how high and bulky in square footage they can be. They determine whether a residential neighborhood will be made up entirely of single-family units or a combination of these and apartments, duplexes, and townhouses. They determine what can go on *in* those buildings—what they can house and what businesses can or cannot operate there—and *on* those buildings (for example, rooftop gardens and greenhouses). And they determine what happens *around* those buildings, too: will a particular neighborhood be housing only, or will schools and businesses be located nearby? Zoning uses both requirements and incentives as its tools for guiding development and construction within cities and city neighborhoods.

The United States' first zoning law was passed in New York City in 1916. In the early twentieth century, zoning was used in the city to ensure that buildings would be set back appropriately from the streets and from each other. Prior to the introduction of these zoning setbacks, New York City streets were constantly dark and damp, with standing water that bred mosquitoes spreading diseases like yellow fever. Zoning setbacks ensured space between buildings to allow air and sunlight to penetrate the streets and dry up those puddles.

Historically, a primary goal of zoning has been to separate housing from everything else, particularly businesses. Indeed, it can be thought of as the process of creating "zones" within cities for different uses. In the era of heavy industrial manufacturing, separating homes from the pollution and noise associated with industry helped to ensure the health of a city's residents. But while the business landscape in many cities has transitioned from manufacturing to retail- and service-oriented businesses, zoning laws are still sometimes used to keep residential neighborhoods purely residential. And we now know that there are repercussions: businesses are unnecessarily separated from their customers, leading to lost opportunities and revenues; the environment suffers owing to an overreliance on automobiles; and those who don't drive must cope with social isolation and dependency when it comes to meeting their most basic needs—which results, in turn, in an increased need for and costs associated with long-term care and supportive services.

And, of course, such antiquated zoning policies have played a hand in creating the food deserts that we find in neighborhoods in too many cities, not to mention contributing to today's epidemics of physical inactivity, obesity, and chronic diseases.

Thankfully, an increasing number of cities are recognizing that these antiquated zoning practices need to be addressed—for the health of our people, our environment, and our businesses. Since zoning is a human-made tool, we can change the rules. We need only realize that times have changed, that our challenges today are different from the challenges of the past, and that zoning rules can be changed to help us successfully conquer today's issues.

When Amanda Burden was appointed commissioner of New York's city planning department in 2002 she began the work of restructuring her department so that it could address the city's twenty-first-century needs. She hired staff members who had fresh ideas and were bold and resolute in their determination to make a difference.

The partnership between the health and city planning departments on the FRESH initiative began with a comparison of data. The health department's yearly Community Health Surveys had shown us where obesity and diabetes rates were highest. We knew, for example, that these diseases were particularly high in our poorest neighborhoods, such as the South Bronx, East and Central Harlem, and North and Central Brooklyn. The health department's studies in these areas had also shown a lack of supermarkets and an abundance of fast food outlets and bode-gas carrying predominantly unhealthy foods and beverages. City Planning maps—compiled using data from the New York State Department of Agriculture and Markets, which licenses and inspects supermarkets—confirmed our findings. When the health department maps were laid on the meeting table next to City Planning's maps of supermarkets (or their lack thereof), the overlap was very nearly a complete match.

Ben Thomases was New York City's first Food Policy Coordinator, and he is a larger-than-life figure with the big talk and big confidence to match his big frame. With his background in business administration, Ben corralled the involved departments into meetings with supermarket owners and operators. The entity in charge of economic development for the city, the NYC Economic Development Corporation (EDC), was also brought onto the working group with the city planning and health departments. We wanted to hear what was preventing the supermarkets from opening stores in our poorest neighborhoods. We asked a simple question: Why aren't you locating in these neighborhoods that need you so badly?

Posing the question directly to supermarket owners revealed that the obstacles were both real and perceived. On the "real" side, the owners told us that the large footprint necessary to achieve the "supermarket" designation made it difficult to open stores in some inner-city locations. Plus, city zoning had stringent requirements for a large number of parking spots with supermarket developments. Owners asked us why this was needed when many of the residents in these neighborhoods didn't even own cars. We confirmed with our data: indeed, car ownership in these poor New York City neighborhoods was low.

City Planning set about addressing the zoning issues. The footprint and parking requirements for supermarkets were both downsized. Once that was achieved, the path to building and opening smaller stores was clear. And the decreased parking would also promote more walking—a win-win, in my estimation.

Next, we turned to the perceived issues. The supermarket operators were convinced they wouldn't be able to make money if they opened stores in poor neighborhoods. "It's going to take too long to break even," they said. "And with all the taxes we have to pay in the state and the city, it's not worth it for us to even try." We thought the owners would be surprised at how well they could do in these neighborhoods, where healthy food choices were so desperately needed, but we clearly needed to offer an incentive. The working group turned to EDC and asked how we might remove these perceived barriers. "We could reduce the tax burden," was one answer that came back. Another was providing tax abatements for mortgages. And maybe we could convince the state to also forgive the sales taxes for equipment and materials needed for supermarket creation and expansion if such construction was occurring in these high-need neighborhoods. Ben Thomases and EDC got to work on the money issues. And so did I.

At around the time of the FRESH discussions and working-group formation, New York State's Department of Health had also issued a request for proposals for chronic disease prevention grants. One of these five-year grants, worth about $80,000 a year, would be enough for us to hire a staff person whose time would be, unlike that of the working group members, devoted entirely to FRESH. With the help of Vicky Grimshaw and Sarah Wolf—my two initial dedicated staff members from the Built Environment and Active Design Program I had started at the city's health department—I rushed to put together a proposal. An initial draft was reviewed and approved by the assistant and deputy commissioners, and then by the health department's grant review committee. On the night before the submission deadline, Vicky, Sarah, and I continued to fine-tune our application as we watched the sky turn its sunset hues of orange and pink before darkening to black. In the morning, with no time to spare for a courier, Vicky boarded an Amtrak train to personally deliver the proposal to the New York State Health Department office in Albany.

A few months later, we learned that our application was successful and we now had the funding to help us hire a dedicated staff person for the implementation of FRESH. And, given the normal delay between job posting and hiring, we also had a few months' worth of dollars accrued from the as-yet-unpaid salary. It was enough to undertake one more thing that Ben Thomases and the working group wanted.

Faced with the supermarket owners' perceived notion that profit could not be made in a poor neighborhood, we'd wished for a way to prove them wrong—to show that they could, indeed, be successful. We'd put out calls for market analysis proposals to show just how many dollars were flowing out of our city and state when people who needed groceries went elsewhere—say, New Jersey—to shop. In these cases, the money these people had for groceries, including food-stamp money, was being lost from city and state tax coffers. What's more, we wondered, wasn't it possible that we could create more jobs in these neighborhoods, where unemployment was high, if we could create or expand supermarkets?

About a year after we'd started work, the pieces of the FRESH initiative had all come together. We had a dedicated coordinator in place and a market leakage analysis report had been completed showing that a lot of money for groceries was flowing out of the city's poorest neighborhoods into places outside the city and even outside the state. People needed groceries and if they couldn't get them in their neighborhoods, they were going elsewhere. EDC had approved mortgage tax abatements and mortgage interest could be tax deducted. The state had agreed to the forgiveness of sales taxes for supermarket construction materials and equipment when such construction occurred in our defined neighborhoods eligible for such FRESH incentives. And City Planning's zoning changes were a done deal. It hadn't been easy, and it hadn't been quick, but through perseverance, cooperation, and creative thinking, we had got the job done.

Today, the FRESH initiative is a decade old and on its fourth full-time coordinator. The New York State Department of Health grant has ended, but, as was my hope and plan, the City has taken up the funding of the coordinator's salary, recognizing that the tax and zoning incentives and resources created for supermarket operators are useful only if someone is dedicated to promoting them to those who need to use them. Since 2008, over twenty supermarkets have been developed or are under development in New York's food deserts. Because the incentives are available *only* for supermarkets located in the neighborhoods that need them, supermarket owners are not able to use them to create stores in areas already rich with such access. Furthermore, because the incentives are tied to the creation of supermarkets with defined spaces and square footages dedicated to fresh foods, FRESH is ensuring access to real food in neighborhoods that were previously deprived. In these stores, at least 30 percent of their space must be dedicated to perishable foods and at least 500 square feet must be given to fresh produce. And the FRESH neighborhoods, also job deserts in many instances, have now seen over a thousand new jobs created. Nearly $100 million of investment has been made in the neighborhoods most in need of economic boosts.

Quenching Our Thirst

Despite all the attention paid to food deserts, it seems we've somehow managed to push the wet stuff to the back of our minds. And yet, the phrase itself almost forces us to remember. After all, in the traditional usage, a "desert" is an area lacking in water.

Clearly, our cities don't have this problem; many, in fact, were intentionally built near sources of water. And yet these same cities sometimes make water a difficult resource for residents to obtain.

Water is the basis of life on earth. Over 70 percent of the Earth's surface is covered with water, and about 60 percent of the human body is made up of the stuff. Without food, we can last around three weeks; without water, we'd likely perish within three days.

Water also happens to be a healthy beverage with zero calories. The fact that so many cities have drinking water that comes straight from a tap is one of the most impressive achievements of the nineteenth and twentieth centuries. Though quality still varies, in much of the developed world, water that comes out of a tap is now largely safe to drink. But strangely, this free, healthy option is increasingly unavailable. When I arrived in New York City in 2006, for example, many school cafeterias didn't serve it, and many daycares didn't provide it. Day in and day out, children learned instead to drink other beverages—many of them high in sugar and bad for their bodies—even as childhood obesity was rapidly increasing.

I knew it didn't have to be this way. I'd traveled to places where I'd seen uniformed schoolchildren filling up their reusable water bottles—some made of stainless steel, some a colorful plastic, some personalized with stickers—at street fountains as they walked home from school. Geneva, for example, has beautiful public fountains: carved bronze lion heads mounted on stone pillars, spouting clean drinking water from their mouths, or big bowls playing host to beautiful sculptures, with water from an adjacent spout designated for drinking. On one memorable visit, I cycled along Lake Geneva admiring the top of Mount Chamonix in nearby France, miraculously visible on that clear day. I knew that free water from the beautiful fountains would be available to quench my thirst as I pedaled the bicycle I'd been able to borrow for free, from one of the kiosks made from modified shipping containers that were found along the dedicated walking and cycling paths surrounding the lake. It was the perfect—and perfectly fitting—end to a trip I'd taken in order to visit colleagues at the World Health Organization to discuss improving our environments globally to prevent chronic diseases like heart disease, diabetes and even some of our most common and deadly cancers such as colon cancer.

On another trip, closer to home, I visited Portland, Oregon. Portland is a city of cyclists—with around 8 percent of the population on two wheels, it has the highest rates of cycling in the United States. But it wasn't the cyclists who caught my eye on this trip; it was the Benson Bubblers.

Simon Benson was born in Norway and moved to Portland in 1879. He got involved in Oregon's main industry, timber, and made millions, which he used to support many philanthropic ventures. Today, a number of Portland amenities are named for him—including the Benson Bubblers. These iconic four-bowl water fountains were installed by the City of Portland in 1912, when Benson donated an amount equivalent to $240,000 in today's dollars. It is said that Benson wanted the twenty or so fountains installed to provide workers with something non-alcoholic to drink during their lunch hour. Another story suggests that he was moved to the gesture after seeing a little girl crying from thirst during a Fourth of July celebration in the city. Whatever the reason, modern-day Portlanders don't have to worry about where their next healthy, thirst-quenching drink is coming from.

In many other cities, New York included, this isn't the case. Easily accessible public drinking water on our city streets and in our workplaces is not so common. As a result, we must either carry our water with us or, more frequently, purchase beverages in small cans or disposable plastic bottles. These many non-biodegradable cans and bottles either enter our increasingly overwhelmed landfills or make their way into the onerous and expensive recycling process. I have seen the mounds of garbage and recycling that pile up each night on New York's city streets; the many empty bottles and cans are easy to spot through the clear recycling bags. Sometimes these purchased beverages are bottled water—not so bad for our health, but not so good for the environment or our wallets. Other times, we're tempted by what first catches our eye in the store (naturally, since they've been placed at eye level): sodas, sweetened iced teas or sports drinks, and other sugar-laden and highly caloric beverages. *This small can of soda can't do too much damage, right?* we think, not realizing that the 250 calories in that drink, ingested daily above and beyond our usual caloric intake, will result in a one-pound weight gain every two weeks—or twenty-six pounds when the year is up. Sometimes we opt for juice, mistakenly thinking it's the healthier choice. Don't be fooled; it too is loaded with unneeded sugar and calories, however natural the sources.

In the years when I was working for the City of New York, Emily Lloyd was the city's commissioner of Environmental Protection. Emily had a clear vision and message about tap water. We must value it. We must preserve it. We should be drinking it. We must improve New Yorkers' access to it. And we must get the public's attention focused on this important issue. During her stint in the post during Mayor Bloomberg's administration, the New York City Department of Environmental Protection introduced Water-on-the-Go.

Picture a typical August afternoon in the city. It's hot, particularly if you've been cycling for miles. This isn't uncommon in the summer, when programs like Summer Streets are in full swing (look for more on Summer Streets in chapter 8). With about seven miles of Park Avenue closed to car traffic on this particular day, many people have come out to ride, or rollerblade, or run, or just to walk. It is late morning and the sun is already unrelenting.

If you brought a water bottle with you when you left home, it's probably been empty for some time. Thankfully, you spy a Water-on-the-Go fountain hooked up to a nearby fire hydrant.

These temporary drinking water stations are popular and well used during summer events. Their high spouts spray cold, cold water into clean white sinks. There's no grimy, clogged drain, and there's no need to put your mouth close to the spout. In fact, the spout is so high that you can easily fill your water bottle.

The Water-on-the-Go fountains are a temporary measure, to be sure, but the initiative provides an example of how we can combat the lack of drinking water access on the streets of our cities. And in New York, more permanent measures are also in the works.

I met Charles McKinney, chief designer for New York City's Department of Parks and Recreation, shortly after I moved to the city in 2006. New York may not feature permanent drinking fountains on its streets, like Geneva or Portland, but it has traditionally provided fountains for the users of its public parks. Between 2006 and 2009, Charles and I worked together on a new water fountain design for the soon-to-open High Line Park (see chapter 8 for more about the High Line). We looked to other cities for inspiration and information, and the health department led focus groups with potential users. We knew that public fountains were often considered "icky," and we wanted to make sure that whatever we ended up building would be used, and not avoided like the plague!

I remember the first time I got a glimpse of the new fountain. Claire Weisz of WXY Studio had come by to present her prototype. It was made of metal, with smooth sloping surfaces for the unused water to trickle down into the ground beneath, watering plants that could be grown around it instead of wasting it in our sewer drains. It had a high spout and no drain, and it could even be programmed to speak or quote poetry from an installed speaker, in keeping with the artistic nature of its setting. "What do you think?" Claire asked. Charles and I looked at each other and smiled. Not only did the fountain look great, but Claire's design avoided the elements that our focus groups had identified as disgusting: clogged drains, low spouts, warm water, and unclean fountain bowls.

The design of the fountain was more than sleek, and more than ick-free—it was functional and low maintenance. The drain-free, clog-free elements meant less need for de-clogging and cleaning, which in turn made the fountains more appealing and more feasible for use in other public areas that had challenges for maintenance. They could potentially be adopted, for example, for the pedestrian plazas being built across the city by New York City's Department of Transportation (DOT); in fact, DOT did agree to include them.

The High Line water fountains were a big step in the right direction, but they were designed for the great outdoors. What about our offices, our public buildings, our schools? By 2010, I had been in New York for more than four years. I had developed great working relationships with colleagues in more than twelve government departments, as well as with many private sector architects, urban planners, developers, and building owners. An opportunity was emerging. The office of Mayor Bloomberg—specifically the Office of Long-Term Planning and Sustainability (OLTPS), which had responsibility for greening the city—was taking on a project to green all construction codes. The zoning codes, the building codes, the plumbing codes, you name it: all were up for reconsideration. The Mayor's Office asked: What could be done with the codes to ensure the improved environmental sustainability of our buildings and their amenities?

The debate about tap water has long been a part of the dialogue about greening and improving our environments. Don't drink bottled water, environmental advocates shout. Although this isn't yet a viable and safe option in substantial areas of the developing world, and sometimes even in some of our communities in the developed world, it is certainly a safe option for most of us who live in the developed world. But viable? Not always. In part, this is a function of accessibility—too few fountains in too few places—but it also comes back to that "ick factor" we dealt with during the High Line fountain design process. Making fountains available is only half of the equation; we have to ensure that people will be willing to use them.

The solution came via a call from Laurie Kerr, the smart-as-a-whip senior policy adviser to OLTPS with whom I'd worked since my move to New York. She was working on proposals for greening the city's plumbing codes. Could we devise some sort of plan for fountains?

Many non-residential buildings, like schools and workplaces, already had water fountains. Usually they were located near the washrooms, where water pipes were in easy proximity for the builders to add this amenity. The problem, though, was the design. Too often, they had low spouts, they had warm water, they had clogged drains if they weren't cleaned frequently. And so, people didn't use them. In this age of bottled and canned beverages, and instant gratification, people also often wanted their drinks sitting conveniently next to them on their desks. Though they might have been willing to refill their bottles or cups every several hours, they weren't necessarily so willing to get up every half hour to take a small sip at the fountain. So, together with Laurie, we came up with a simple yet elegant idea: the addition of water bottle refilling stations.

Imagine not having to put your mouth close to a spout at all. Imagine just holding your reusable water bottle under a tap— one that's not in a bathroom—and filling it with water that you could drink at your own pace at your desk, or in the boardroom, or in a colleague's office. This, then, would become the basis for improving tap water access within buildings in New York.

Packaged with a whole host of other, more complicated changes, the idea soon passed City Council's vote. And voilà, all building construction from this point on would include water bottle refilling stations with their already previously-mandated drinking water fountains. No more "ick factor" for workers who wanted to drink tap water during the work day. Drinking tap water rather than sugar-sweetened beverages from the vending machine would finally become a truly viable choice. Sometimes, policy change can be that simple, when you have the right partnerships.

On the Road

Better bodegas, Health Bucks, FRESH, Water-on-the Go: the types of partnerships that result in these initiatives—in which multiple government departments cooperate both with each other and with the private sector to provide access to previously unavailable or unaffordable healthy choices—are a success story that's spreading around the world.

Like me, Lyn James is a public health doctor. Also like me, she worked for the Epidemic Intelligence Service at the U.S. Centers for Disease Control and Prevention. In fact, that's where Lyn and I met. Unlike me, though, Lyn chose to do her work as a disease detective in Chicago's Department of Public Health. Braving the cold, biting winters, Lyn focused on infectious disease issues in the Windy City. This was an especially brave choice, since Lyn had moved there from the tropical, humid heat of Singapore. The Singaporean government had agreed to grant Lyn a two-year hiatus from her position there on the condition that she return to share any new knowledge and skills she had gained from her experience in the United States. And so, in 2006, while I was making my way to New York, Lyn returned home to head the Singapore Ministry of Health's group working on infectious disease epidemiology. It was a great and welcome surprise to me to discover that

Lyn had transitioned to leading Singapore's chronic disease prevention team by the time I decided to visit her in February 2013.

On a hot, clear, sunny Saturday in Singapore, Lyn picked me up in her little two-door car and whisked me off to a "hawkers' center" for lunch. A hawkers' center is a food court of sorts: small carts owned by different vendors are spread throughout the location, some under cover of a roof and protected by walls, and others open to the elements. Hawkers' centers are also popular eating spots in Malaysia, where the locals love to dine out first thing in the morning before work, during the lunch break, for dinner, or for late after-dinner meals. Local food is cheap and affordable, and it's delicious. For less than one American or Canadian dollar, you can buy a plate of stir-fried noodles with eggs, crispy pork rinds, and bean sprouts; a bowl of umpteen varieties of noodle soup; thick coconut curries; or tamarind- and seafood-infused soups. The list goes on and on. The mix of cultures in Malaysia and Singapore has spawned a cuisine with Chinese, Thai, Malay, and Indian influences. It's as easy to get Chinese noodles as it is to find Indian rotis and Malay rice dishes with curry.

Just a few days earlier, I'd visited a hawkers' center in Kuala Lumpur, where I had gone, on behalf of the World Health Organization, to scout possible case studies of healthy built-environment intervention projects for physical activity. I had been picked up at the airport by my cousin Nick, his wife, Pauline, and their two adult sons, Jonathan and Justin. On the way home—at 11:00 p.m.—we'd stopped at a hawkers' center for a snack. Despite the late hour on a weeknight, the parking lot was almost full. Many tables, both inside and out, were occupied. We opted for outside and pulled red plastic chairs up to a round table topped with scuffed wood laminate. As we took our seats, a waiter appeared to take our order for drinks. Recalling the travel advisories about avoiding ice, I asked for hot water with lemon and was met with a blank stare. I ordered hot Ovaltine instead, hoping the chocolaty drink would be lower in caffeine than the tea and coffee also available. Nick ordered sweet tea, Pauline settled on iced coffee, and their two sons chose sodas. They also ordered a variety of rotis and dipping curries, which arrived quickly. Pauline suggested that I try the rotis, telling me that one in particular was "good" for me; it was made from whole wheat rather than white flour. I dipped the bread into one of the curry sauces and put the delicious morsel in my mouth. It might have been made from wheat flour, but I couldn't help but notice the generous amount of butter spread on it. I wondered what else was inside, and what the calorie and fat content might be.

In Singapore, Lyn promised me a different experience. She was about to serve as my tour guide to one of the "healthy" hawkers' centers created with the help of the Singaporean government. Recognizing that so many people in Singapore eat out—and eat out extensively at hawkers' centers—the Singaporean government decided to do what it could to increase healthy choices for consumers at these venues. Food safety is also paramount at the centers, and the government regularly inspects for food safety measures.

The first thing I noticed was the greater number of stalls here than at the smaller center I'd visited on my first night in Kuala Lumpur. On our initial walk-through, Lyn pointed out some of the features of her government's initiative: options for regular noodles or whole wheat; the government-issued signs with logos designating a vendor who had opted to participate in the healthy hawkers' initiative by changing the fats or oils used in cooking, or offering healthier alternatives such as whole-grain noodles along with the more refined varieties. Ready to eat, I opted for char kway teow—flat rice noodles stir-fried with eggs, chili, bean sprouts, and Chinese chives—with extra bean sprouts, minus the shrimp (I'm allergic), and Chinese sausage. I purchased this from a "healthy vendor," easily identified by the logo of the Singaporean government's initiative. It was good to know, as I savored the delicious dish, that the vendor had left out the artery-clogging pork fat commonly used.

For initiatives such as this one, Singapore's Ministry of Health funds and works closely with an organization called the Health Promotion Board. The field of health promotion was formalized in 1986 with the ratification of the Ottawa Charter for Health Promotion, which encouraged signatories to promote health and well-being using five main methods: reorienting health services, helping people develop personal skills, strengthening community action, creating more supportive environments, and building healthy public policies. Though initially adopted in Ottawa, the charter, unfortunately for Canadians, is too often cited and not often enough implemented comprehensively in Canada. Since 1986, Canada has fallen behind many other countries that have seriously taken on the comprehensive work of health promotion. In Singapore, as in Canada and the United States and most countries now around the world, chronic diseases such as heart disease and stroke are the leading causes of death. The government in Singapore, in tandem with the Health Promotion Board, is working hard to address the risk factors for these diseases, including, of course, unhealthy diets.

As Lyn and I ate, we spoke about how the government was making it feasible for vendors to procure healthier ingredients affordably. I asked if the whole wheat noodles and healthier fats used were the same price as the more commonly used, less healthy ingredients.

"They are now," Lyn answered, "thanks to the government's interference."

Lyn explained that the government acts as a go-between for the sale of the ingredients. The vendors in the hawkers' center are small, and on their own few can afford to buy the whole wheat noodles or healthier oils in the large quantities needed for lower prices. With the government's help, orders from multiple vendors can be coordinated and wholesale prices secured. It's a system that has benefited the vendors and the suppliers, and provided consumers with healthier choices.

I nodded as Lyn talked, recognizing the hard work, creative thinking, and cooperation that had gone into this program. Like the changes we'd undertaken back in New York, the healthy hawkers' initiative was born out of a desire and necessity for change coupled with outside-the-box thinking, hard work, and a boatload of cooperation. It too relied on a combination of public education, government intervention, and private-sector involvement. And like those changes closer to home, it was a living demonstration of the fact that we can, indeed, change for the better how we eat. When it comes to the fight against obesity and its many consequences, that definitely is a step in the right direction.

3 | AN EARLY START

INOCULATING FOR OBESITY IN SCHOOLS AND DAYCARES

WE'VE TALKED A LOT now about improving the landscape when it comes to healthy food choices and affordability. But many of the policy and mindset shifts we've explored take something for granted: that the people who stand to be positively impacted by these initiatives are willing and able to make their own decisions concerning what they put in their mouths. What happens, though, if that's not the case? What about our kids?

It is now a known fact that obese children grow up to be obese adults. That's a dire situation, and it's not even the whole story. Obese children are not waiting until adulthood to develop the serious health repercussions associated with obesity. Diseases that were once considered a problem only beginning in middle age—such as type 2 diabetes, high blood pressure, and high cholesterol—are now showing up in our children.

In 1997, during my second year of medical school, I learned that type 2 diabetes was also referred to as adult-onset diabetes. Not any more. Two decades on, the medical profession has dropped "adult-onset" because it no longer applies. Pediatricians report seeing the disease in teenagers and children in increasing numbers. Why? Because of obesity. We are no longer just a generation of unhealthy adults; that same unhealthiness is evident in our kids.

The impending societal consequences are mind-boggling. Medical complications from conditions like type 2 diabetes, high blood pressure, and high cholesterol that once made their first appearance in old age—a decade or two after diagnosis—will start to show themselves when our children reach their teens and early adulthood. Complications like heart attacks and strokes. Complications of diabetes like blindness, limb amputations, and kidney failure requiring dialysis or transplant. This could happen before our boys become men, before our girls become women. It's a bleak picture, no doubt. But unless something changes— and soon—it will be our reality.

FitnessGram: An Important First Step

It has long been a practice of schools to ensure that children like little Peggy Ann McKay—star of Shel Silverstein's well-known poem "Sick"—are kept home from school. Poor Peggy Ann, with her alarming list of ailments, including "measles and the mumps / A gash, a rash and purple bumps"! The practice of infection control has always been a priority for the school system: notes are sent imploring parents to keep sick children home; phone calls are made to come pick up a child who is not feeling well. Today, schools also routinely check vaccination records before permitting a child to attend classes. In Canada, some provinces, such as Ontario, Manitoba, and New Brunswick, have made up-to-date vaccinations a requirement for attending school. This support for and encouragement of inoculation has been incredibly successful in making what used to be common childhood diseases relatively rare. Measles comes with a 1-in-1,000 chance of permanent brain damage as a complication, and before the dawning of the age of inoculation, when practically every child had measles at some point or another, this was far from unheard-of. Now, with immunizations common among children, few get such diseases—and fewer still suffer the serious and preventable consequences.

Checking for childhood vaccination at school entry means that vaccination rates are known and tracked, and public health departments know a great deal about vaccination rates for infectious diseases. Unfortunately, the same can't be said when it comes to gathering knowledge about non-communicable diseases such as obesity. When I arrived in New York in 2006, precious little was known about the rates of childhood obesity. Because this information was largely unmeasured and untracked, what small bits of knowledge we could glean about this epidemic came from rare individual studies. One, published in 2003, a one-time study of elementary school children in kindergarten to grade five, showed that only about half were at a healthy weight. Another study, published in 2006 and focused on children between the ages of two and four enrolled in the state's Head Start programs, found that 42 percent of these very young children were already overweight or obese. It was useful information to have, but nowhere near complete. What was happening to our children in school in middle school and high school? What were the trends over time, even in our elementary schools? We didn't know—but we needed to. The first step in mounting any type of attack is to gather knowledge. We had none.

It was with this urgency that I boarded a plane for Dallas, Texas, soon after starting my work in New York City. Once on the ground, I rolled my scuffed carry-on through the airport on a quest for the car rental booth, thinking that I really did need to get a new suitcase. I hadn't expected to travel much as a local government employee, but my New York colleagues and I were often invited to national meetings because of the innovative work we were undertaking, and many of our local initiatives were hailed as examples for national and even international dissemination and adoption. I made my way down the long airport corridors, opting to walk beside the moving sidewalks instead of on them— an attempt to log a few steps on my pedometer before sitting in a car for several hours.

I picked up my four-door sedan, armed myself with a map (these were the days before GPS), and began the drive to the resort where the Cooper Institute meeting was taking place. Founded in 1970 by Dr. Kenneth H. Cooper—popularly known as the "father of aerobics"—the Cooper Institute is a non-profit group with the mission of promoting health and wellness through exercise. One of the Institute's accomplishments was the development of a children's weight and fitness assessment to help schools improve their physical education programs, a system known as FitnessGram. It was FitnessGram that we were meeting to discuss.

The weather in Dallas was foggy and rainy, and I sighed with relief when I finally pulled into the parking lot of a hotel that resembled a giant log cabin. Not long after I checked in, I heard someone call my name. I turned around to see David Freedman, a colleague from my time with the CDC. I smiled at the sight of him, dressed in his usual loose-fitting T-shirt, beige khaki pants, and Birkenstock sandals. He told me he was at the FitnessGram meeting to present the CDC's case in support of more systematic and consistent methods of evaluating childhood obesity in school-children. I was there to present on the same issue. Once again, it seemed, we were allies in a common cause.

To understand the excitement of public health practitioners about FitnessGram, it's important to remember that no reliable and consistent weight-related statistics were being gathered in schools at the time. While some schools were indeed gathering information, it was scattershot at best. Weight might be taken, but not height. A scale might be used, or perhaps calipers to measure skinfolds and fat levels. And there was no attempt to track changes over time.

FitnessGram represented an effort to improve on that model. The tool allowed children to be consistently measured using their weight and height, and it facilitated a comparison of their body mass index (BMI) percentile to statistics gathered in the 1960s, before the obesity epidemic took hold. Another option for measurement prior to the Dallas meeting was through the use of skin calipers. The key issue was the accurate use of skin calipers that would have required extensive training for school staff, and it would have taken much too long to assess the more than one million New York City public schoolchildren. Using one method—weight and height measurement—consistently across the board would yield the least confusing, most meaningful data. By the time of the Cooper Institute gathering, FitnessGram was already being used in more and more states. David and the CDC wanted to make sure the trend continued, and so did I. FitnessGram represented our best hope for gathering the data we'd need to truly track and combat the childhood obesity epidemic.

As the two-day meeting wrapped up, a consensus was beginning to emerge about the consistent use of weight and height measurements and BMI percentile to track children's weights over time, rather than skinfold measurements. It was an important step, and I was thrilled to head back to New York with the good news.

In the wake of the Cooper Institute meeting, the adoption of FitnessGram moved full-speed ahead in New York City public schools. Children from kindergarten to grade twelve would be measured every school year with the tool. Older children, those above grade five, would also have their fitness levels measured by a series of tests in physical education classes. The Office of School Health, whose assistant commissioner reported to both the Department of Health and Mental Hygiene, and the Education Department, was called upon to work with both to implement this initiative.

Devices to measure weight and height were purchased and shipped out to public schools. School staff was trained to measure children's weights and heights and plot them on the supplied BMI percentile charts. The data would be sent to the Education Department and Office of School Health for analysis and tabulation. And public school children in New York City would be sent home with FitnessGram report cards.

Yup. A report card, just the like ones we're so used to seeing for academic achievement. This was new, to be sure, and it no doubt took some getting used to. Picture this: Johnny comes home from school on report card day, excited to share his progress with his parents. Mom and Dad are surprised to see not one but two reports this time around. The FitnessGram report card is something they haven't encountered during Johnny's first three years in elementary school. His mother now recalls a letter sent home from the school, introducing the new program. She and Johnny's father look at the report after dinner as Johnny sits on the living room floor, doing his schoolwork. They're alarmed to see that their son falls into the red zone, rather than the yellow or green zone, on the sheet Johnny's mother now has on her lap. Johnny's mother reads the instructions suggesting that they take Johnny to his pediatrician or family doctor for assessment, since he falls in the obese category based on the FitnessGram screening measurements done at school. She flips the page over to see if there's anything more. Indeed there is: instructions to limit his TV watching to less than two hours a day, and to ensure he gets at least sixty minutes of moderate- to vigorous-intensity physical activity daily. There are also recommendations for a healthier diet—including eating more vegetables and fruits, drinking water, avoiding sugar-sweetened beverages, and limiting juice. Ideas for what the family can do to be more active are also included. "Put on some music and dance" is among the suggestions that need not cost the family any money, assuming there's a radio or stereo at home. Johnny's mother makes a mental note to stop buying soda and juice drinks, and to start serving water at dinner. *Johnny really does watch way too much TV*, she thinks to herself.

The adoption of the FitnessGram assessment tool was a game-changer. For the first time, parents were made aware of whether their child's weight was healthy. If the child fell into the green zone, all was well. The yellow zone indicated some cause for concern: the child was possibly overweight. The red zone suggested that the child was likely obese, and at risk for serious health issues. The advice to limit TV, eat and drink more healthily, and get sixty minutes of daily physical activity was intended for all families, so that even children at a healthy weight would have support in maintaining that over time. Parents of children in the yellow and red zones were advised to see their doctors to confirm their children's weight status and to discuss their children's health.

For some, it was a rude awakening—parents love to think that their children are perfect. But it's more important to have the full picture, to know if a child's weight is unhealthy and their overall health at risk. It's equally important to know that it's never too late to intervene, and that even small and simple changes can make a big difference.

In 2011, a few years after the FitnessGram rollout, I invited Arkansas's surgeon general, Dr. Joseph Thompson, to be a keynote speaker at our Fit City conference in New York City (see chapter 4 for more on Fit City conferences). Arkansas was among the first states to measure children's weights and heights in school. Dr. Thompson, a young and young-at-heart pediatrician, had been an early proponent of using childhood obesity measurement and report cards to address the epidemic in his state. We'd first met at a Maine Heart Foundation conference, where the good doctor could be found dancing up a storm at the evening reception after a long day of presentations, including his own! In recognition of their successes in addressing childhood obesity, Dr. Thompson and his team would eventually win a Translating Research to Policy Award, conferred at the Active Living Research Conference. Dr. Thompson had found that measuring the weights of schoolchildren and arming their parents with those report cards made a difference. Arkansas showed one of the earliest reversals in childhood obesity in North America.

FitnessGram increased our awareness in other crucial ways as well. For New York City's Department of Health and Mental Hygiene, and its public schools, analyses of the data confirmed the results of earlier studies conducted on children in the city between three and five years old, and also on two-year-olds, that suggested many New York City kids were overweight or obese. The data also showed that kids with poor fitness levels were not doing as well academically as their more fit classmates. As follow-up occurred over time, a pattern emerged: children who got fitter also improved academically. These longitudinal studies constitute rare evidence of possible causal relationships between fitness and academics/school performance. Like the parents who'd received the FitnessGram report cards, the schools realized that they had to do more to deal with the issue of childhood fitness and obesity.

The partnership between the Department of Health and Mental Hygiene and the Education Department in New York has led to many fruitful initiatives—literally. Salad bars were introduced into middle and high schools. Water coolers were placed in school lunch lines so children could fill their cups with this calorie-free, healthy drink. The initial piloting of these initiatives in some schools in the highest-needs neighborhoods, with the highest rates of obesity, showed that the interventions could work across all schools. Their eventual system-wide implementation meant that all kids in New York would benefit. Along with Arkansas,

New York City is among the first jurisdictions to show reversals in childhood obesity trends.

Beyond the Schoolyard

Addressing the issue of what kids are offered to eat within schools is vital, but what happens once they step off school grounds? What happens when they head to the convenience stores and fast food outlets that are all too easily accessible on lunch breaks or on the way home?

Much more discussion is needed about the food environments around schools. Studies done in the United States show that children are consuming about 10 to 15 percent of their daily total calories from sugar-sweetened beverages. Cities such as New York and Toronto have worked to encourage bodega and convenience store owners to offer healthy alternatives, but it's not enough: junk food is still readily available, and often placed in the most enticing spots. All too frequently, fast food outlets are found within walking distance of schools, tempting our kids with a convenient spot to hang out and consume sweet, salty, and fatty treats that are affordable even on a small allowance. No wonder fast food outlets and convenience stores often spring up around schools: they can rely on a flow of minors to buy their high-calorie, nutrient-poor offerings on a regular basis.

Some cities, however, have said enough is enough. Years ago, many cities passed zoning laws banning the sale of alcohol near schools. Now, using zoning laws to get the job done, Detroit has banned fast food restaurants from locating within five hundred feet of a school.

Before It's Too Late

The efforts made to address obesity-related issues among school-age children are a good start, but they are just a start. Given the studies showing that nearly half of children as young as age two are already overweight or obese, school interventions may be coming too late for many kids. The health department realized it could—and needed to—improve healthy opportunities for younger children as well.

Early on in the Bloomberg administration, the New York City Department of Health and Mental Hygiene decided that it would use its administrative and legal powers to tackle the epidemics of obesity and diabetes where it could. When it came to many aspects of the physical environment—such as the design and construction of our buildings, streets, and neighborhoods— the Department of Health and Mental Hygiene itself had no direct jurisdiction, so interventions in these areas would require partnerships with other government departments and private-sector players. There were, however, two main settings that were regulated and inspected by the health department. The first, restaurants, was the focus of our calorie-labeling initiative (discussed in chapter 1). A second key setting was daycares.

Daycares in urban settings are generally inspected by environmental health officers or inspectors working for the departments of health or public health. Because inspectors routinely visit these establishments, they are able to ensure that laws and regulations are being enforced. In the same way that health inspectors were able to efficiently combine inspection visits to restaurants with monitoring of compliance with calorie-labeling laws, the health department's goal was to utilize its inspectors to monitor compliance with daycare regulations. But first, the city had to have new daycare regulations for obesity to enforce!

Lynn Silver, a New York City assistant commissioner for Chronic Disease Prevention and Control, was a woman on a mission. After many years away on the faculty at a university in Brazil, and a short stint as a fellow at Sweden's Karolinska Institute, a research-led medical university, Lynn was now back in New York, and she immediately got to work. Like me, Lynn wanted to apply legal methods that had been used in the past for infectious diseases to control and prevent today's most salient non-communicable health problems. And because these health problems—particularly obesity, type 2 diabetes, high blood pressure, and high cholesterol—were now increasingly seen in our children, preventing and controlling the obesity epidemic in children became a mainstay of her work, and mine.

A visit to a New York City daycare in the late 1990s or early 2000s likely would have revealed practices that would seem pretty unhealthy compared to New York City's standards today. In some daycares, juice drinks loaded with sugar were on offer throughout the day, with no limits, and water simply wasn't provided. Kids could be found sitting in front of TVs, their eyes glued to the screen and their bodies motionless, sometimes for prolonged periods. Of course, some daycares were better than others. The question was how to make *all* daycares as good as the best ones, especially for these littlest members of our society who couldn't speak up for themselves.

We set our sights on enforceable and consistent standards. The health department established standards for foods and beverages. No more sugar-sweetened drinks. Children could have juice but with limits, since even juices with a 100 percent fruit content are very high in sugar. Daycares would be required to put jugs of water out so children could drink water throughout the day, whenever they got thirsty. And unlimited TV watching would be a thing of the past. Television viewing was still permitted, but only for an hour each day, and only quality educational programs. To fill up those hours that had been spent in front of a screen, daycares needed to get their children physically active—at the very least, for the sixty minutes each day recommended by the U.S. Department of Health and Human Services Physical Activity Guidelines. These standards were drafted by the Department of Health and Mental Hygiene, and brought to the Board of Health, which governs the health department's activities and regulations. The board voted to establish these standards in 2006. They understood that our youngest children needed them, and that we as a city had a responsibility to provide healthy choices—and remove unhealthy ones—when parents weren't around. In other words, the options made available to our young children had to default to healthy alternatives.

In 2014, several authors published a paper in the journal *Preventing Chronic Disease* on the effects of new daycare regulations on the health of New York City children. The study team visited 106 daycares, each on two consecutive days, for four hours, to collect data on a total of 636 children. Among the successes found in the study was improvement in children's consumption of healthy beverages, and a decrease in the consumption of less-healthy choices.

PART TWO

HOW WE BUILD

Today, we spend the vast majority of our time in buildings. And the vast majority of *that* time is, unfortunately, sedentary. We sit on couches and at desks. We take elevators and escalators. We skip our lunch breaks to get one more memo written, or our early-morning fitness class in favor of an extra hour of sleep. No one's denying that sleep is a good thing, or that the memo really needed to be written, but all of that sitting? Well, that's definitely bad.

For quite some time, we've known that regular bouts of physical activity are important for health. But recent studies are revealing that decreasing sedentariness in our daily lives is also important. A 2013 Norwegian study compared the impacts of physical activity and sedentariness on health-related parameters in healthy adults. The researchers found that while moderate- to vigorous-intensity physical activity was associated with increased HDL ("good" cholesterol), sedentary behavior was associated with increased LDL ("bad" cholesterol) and triglycerides (unhealthy fats in the blood). In other words, both moderate- to vigorous-intensity physical activity *and* decreased levels of sedentariness appeared to be important for optimizing health. In 2015, a Swedish study looked at the association of metabolic syndrome—a cluster of conditions that increase one's risk of heart disease, stroke, and diabetes—with physical activity and sedentary behavior. This study found that time spent sedentary doubled the odds of metabolic syndrome, while cardiorespiratory fitness, moderate- to vigorous-intensity physical activity, and even light-intensity physical activity decreased the odds of metabolic syndrome.

Today, metabolic syndrome is said to afflict some 47 million Americans, or over 15 percent of the U.S. population. That means that more than 15 percent of the U.S. population is afflicted concurrently with at least three of these five risk factors: high blood pressure, high blood sugar, low "good" cholesterol, high triglycerides, and large waist size. Those who have this triad of factors are at a much greater risk than those who do not for heart disease, stroke, and diabetes. Helping people to increase their regular physical activity *and* decrease their sedentariness is more important than ever.

So, what do our buildings have to do with all of this? A lot, as it turns out.

When it comes to the different strategies that have been employed to encourage people to both increase moderate- to vigorous-intensity physical activity and decrease sedentariness, our buildings and their designs can play a critical role. For example, buildings can be designed to enable and encourage daily stair climbing among those able to do so. Our buildings and their amenities can be designed to increase bouts of standing and moving rather than sitting. Our buildings can be designed to provide opportunities for convenient and easy intentional— and unintentional—exercise during the workday, or once we are at home.

And just what can these small bouts of activity do? Calculations by physical activity experts suggest that a mere *two minutes* of additional stair climbing each day would burn sufficient calories to prevent the annual average weight gains currently seen in adults. Another study—in which ten thousand Harvard alumni men were followed over a thirteen-year period—found that the men who reported climbing twenty to thirty-four floors of stairs per week (that's the equivalent to three to five floors per day) showed a 29 percent reduction in their risk of stroke—independent of whether or not these men exercised in their leisure time.

So, we can keep on building in the style of recent decades, and keep watching our health decline, or we can start building smart, by building active. In fact, this way of thinking about building might take us back to the old days, before we could count on fast elevators and lots of escalators!

4 | ACTIVE DESIGN

THE BIRTH OF A MOVEMENT

The journey of a thousand miles begins with a single step.

—LAO TZU, *Tao Te Ching*

I like to see myself as a bridge builder, that is me building bridges between people, between races, between cultures, between politics, trying to find common ground.

—T.D. JAKES

I LOVE THE APPLE STORE on Fifth Avenue in New York City. Sure, the sleek and shiny technology is fun to look at and play with, and the resident "geniuses" are always incredibly friendly, but the store itself is the real draw. It's situated smack in the middle of General Motors Plaza, or *under* GM Plaza, to be precise. The ground-level atrium is enclosed by a stunning glass cube, unsupported by steel, that reaches more than thirty feet into the sky. It's amazing, no doubt. But the thing that gets me, every single time, is the spiral glass staircase. It greets you as soon as you step inside. Your eyes are immediately drawn to it—and so, it turns out, are your feet. In my experience (and you bet I've stood and watched!), people are generally halfway down that flight of stairs before they even realize that a glass elevator is neatly tucked into the center of the staircase. In this particular store, out of sight is clearly out of mind.

The store opened in May 2006, just before I moved to New York. Its design got a lot of attention, but not everything inside those glass walls was unique. The prominent staircase that had caught my attention was, it turned out, an iconic Apple Store feature. The company's first retail shop in New York—located in a former post office building in SoHo—had sported one as early as 2002. These days, they can be found all over the world—in London, Paris, Tokyo, and beyond.

I know. You're reading this and wondering, what's so darn exciting about a staircase, right? Well, if you spend a good portion of your life trying to figure out ways to encourage people to be more active, then staircases are a hot topic—especially staircases that make you forget that elevators even exist. These days, the thinking that goes into the decision to prioritize a staircase and all but hide an elevator is called Active Design. But back in the early 2000s, when Apple was building those stores, the concept was still unheard-of. Apple was ahead of the curve—unintentionally, because its designers and builders were more concerned with aesthetics than health—but by the time I landed in New York in June 2006, I was working hard to catch up.

Fit City 1: The Brainstorming Begins

Although I didn't know it at the time, my earliest work on behalf of the New York City Department of Health and Mental Hygiene would lead—eventually—to the birth of the Active Design movement.

I had accepted Lynn Silver's offer to join New York's Bureau of Chronic Disease Prevention and Control as deputy to the assistant commissioner, and while I was still in Atlanta, wrapping up my time at the CDC, Lynn and I were discussing the best way to launch our efforts around the built environment and health. One of the many ideas we kicked around was a brainstorming conference—one that would bring together different disciplines to start a conversation about health. Lynn then introduced me to Rick Bell. Rick was an architect, a former assistant commissioner at the New York City Department of Design and Construction (DDC), and the executive director of the New York chapter of the American Institute of Architects (AIANY). It made strategic sense for us to work together. AIANY was in a position to reach the groups we wanted to reach if we were going to improve the designs of our spaces for health: the architects and urban designers responsible for our buildings, streets, and neighborhoods.

AIANY is housed in the Center for Architecture, a combination office, exhibition, and education space southwest of Washington Square Park, where continuing-education programs are offered to architects, landscape architects, urban designers, and the public. When we managed to connect by phone, Rick told me how the center had recently mounted an obesity exhibit, in which an artist had used brightly colored soda cans to represent rates of obesity across the country. Picture a map of the United States with the states represented by cans of different colors—blue for states with rates of obesity below 20 percent, yellow for those between 20 and 25 percent, orange for those between 25 and 30 percent, and fire-engine red for those states with the highest rates of obesity, above 30 percent. I was surprised—I hadn't expected a group of architects to be concerned about the same modern-day epidemics that kept me busy in my day-to-day work. But Rick's wife was a pediatrician, so he was well aware of just how damaging our rising obesity rates were. Rick was on board with our idea for a brainstorming event, and over the next six months we would speak biweekly, then in weekly conference calls, to mount the inaugural Fit City conference.

My first "in person" duty on the job in New York was to attend what came to be called "Fit City 1," the conference Rick and I had been planning for six months. At around 8:00 a.m. on a warm but rainy weekday, conference attendees—a combination of health professionals, design and planning professionals, city staff from various departments, and even interested members of the public—began to trickle into AIANY's main conference space, two floors below the entrance level but still flooded with natural light thanks to the building's open-concept design. After helping ourselves to a healthy breakfast and a cup of coffee or tea, we found our way to our seats to eat and listen. Rick stepped to the podium to begin introductions. The lights were dimmed, and the image projected on the large white wall behind him came into focus, showing the staircase we had just descended, with its vibrant orange-red railings, contrasting with its walls painted white. And on the slide, the words "FIT CITY" were in black in the bottom left corner. AIANY had deliberately used an image of its own staircase in the poster for the conference. The center was proud of the fact that most people who entered the building on the first floor and descended to the second or third floors below—and then back up again—almost always did so via the stairs. Magnetic devices held open the doors leading to the stairway (though they would demagnetize and close for safety reasons in the event of a fire), and that vibrant orange-red solid railing drew the eye toward the stairs rather than the elevator, whose doors were painted to blend in with the surrounding white walls. Though not yet generally allowed in 2006 in New York City's building codes, AIANY had asked for an exception to be granted from the Department of Buildings to allow the use of the magnetic devices. So, when visitors arrived at the center and made their way downstairs, Rick would often proudly ask if they'd even noticed the elevator. I hadn't—at least not until he'd pointed it out.

Rick and I had arranged for New York City Health Commissioner Tom Frieden to open the conference. Not having met Tom yet in person, I recall being surprised when he stood up from his chair and made his way to the podium. His slight frame stood in contrast to his larger-than-life reputation. By 2006, Tom had already made a name for himself in the public health world for successfully reducing rates in smoking in Mayor Bloomberg's New York through many new policies, including smoke-free laws, higher taxes, and hard-hitting ads. The successes in New York City had in turn inspired many other cities and countries around the world to enact such measures. And prior to the successes in tobacco control, Tom had already distinguished himself as the key person introducing vigorous review processes aimed at controlling the growing, multi-drug-resistant TB problem in New York City.

Tom's confident and authoritative voice is one that quickly commands attention. At Fit City 1, he began by presenting the slides that I had created for him. He flashed Lynn's favorite images—the CDC obesity maps, changing increasingly from blue to yellow to orange to red with each passing year since the mid 1980s. As Tom clicked through each year from 1985 through 2005, we watched as the colors changed in more and more states, representing rising obesity rates. And yes, there was West Virginia in red, indicating rates of adult obesity above 30 percent. Tom stressed that obesity and diabetes were the two health problems in New York City that were getting worse, not better. Infectious diseases were well controlled, and smoking rates were declining thanks to the health department's recent efforts. But obesity and diabetes were heading in the other direction.

I think I spent as much time watching the audience as I did watching Tom. From my seat at the front of the room, I would periodically turn around to glance at the size of the crowd and gauge reactions. I was tense at first. The seats were not fully filled when Tom began, but as his lecture proceeded, the fashionably late started to file in. In the end, the AIANY staff managing the sign-in table tallied about 150 people. Not a bad start, and certainly an indication of interest in what we were trying to do.

Back at the podium, Tom was followed by the CDC's Dr. Candace Rutt. I had invited Candace to attend back when we were still analyzing our community walkability data from West Virginia. Her role was to reinforce the commissioner's message, and to present evidence showing that the built environment could be a major factor in increasing physical activity.

The list of presenters that first year was impressive. Dr. Mindy Fullilove, a psychiatrist from Columbia University's Mailman School of Public Health, spoke about the importance of connecting people from different neighborhoods, and the ways in which parks can help to do this. Multiple architects, urban planners, and accessibility experts shared their ideas. Among them were architect Linda Pollak, with whom I'd end up working on library and pedestrian plaza projects in Queens; Ronnette Riley, the award-winning architect of the SoHo Apple Store, with its iconic staircase; Rob Lane from the Regional Plan Association, who spoke about the NYC Quality Housing Initiative; Matt Urbanski, landscape architect, who addressed the importance of integrating active recreation opportunities into everyday life; Hillary Brown, architect; and Matt Sapolin, commissioner of the Mayor's Office for People with Disabilities, who spoke of creating active opportunities for all through building and site opportunities such as ramps. Dr. Richard Jackson, former director of the National Center for Environmental Health at the CDC, then on the faculty at the University of California–Berkeley, presented the closing keynote address, reiterating what Tom and Candace had said earlier. The message was loud and clear: we had an obesity epidemic on our hands, it was getting worse, and there were things we could do in terms of our built environment that had the potential to make it better.

That concluded the public part of the program. The afternoon session would be for the speakers and the City department staff in attendance. People seemed excited . . . and hungry!

In the library space on the center's main floor we grabbed a sandwich and salad and took our places around a very large conference table. After Rick thanked everyone for coming, we went around the table and introduced ourselves and our job responsibilities; AIANY had done well in getting a variety of New York City department staff to attend both the conference and the lunch discussion. There were people attending from departments we needed to engage, such as the Departments of Buildings, Transportation, and Parks and Recreation. Our session turned to working our way down a list of questions that I'd prepared for the participants, to stimulate discussion and elicit ideas about what we should do next in the city. For example, we asked participants to identify what we could get started on within their own departments, a month or week or day after the conference.

The first Fit City Conference was over, but the ideas it generated would create a new movement. And interest in our initiative kept growing, with the number of annual attendees rising to more than four hundred, so that in 2014 we had to move the conference to a bigger venue, an auditorium at The New School.

Getting to Know LEED

Follow-up to Fit City 1 began almost immediately. I met with Deborah Taylor, an architect who'd attended as a representative of the New York City Department of Buildings. At the conference luncheon, where we'd met, Deborah had told the group that she was working hard on "greening" the city's buildings. For example, the City was looking at how all construction codes, from building codes to plumbing codes, could be used to improve the environment. It was Deborah's job at the Department of Buildings to work with the Mayor's Office of Long-Term Planning and Sustainability to address those items that could be improved specifically for and in our building codes. How could building warming and cooling systems be made more efficient? How could we decrease the air pollutants emitted from buildings? How could our buildings save electricity? How could we ensure we wasted less water? Deborah immediately raised an interesting idea: perhaps, alongside the greening initiatives, health initiatives could also be integrated into building design. In fact, maybe the two initiatives could even be pursued concurrently.

And so, on one of my first days as an official resident of New York City, Deborah, Lynn Silver, and I met for lunch. Deborah told us about a recently passed law that required all city construction—new builds as well as major renovations—to be "green" starting in 2007. For many buildings, particularly office and institutional sites, that green designation would be achieved by LEED certification at the silver level. At that point in my career, I'd never heard of LEED, but I was curious to know more. Deborah made sure I had all the information I needed, and I got busy bringing myself up to speed.

LEED—or Leadership for Energy and Environmental Design—is a certification program that was created in the early 2000s by the non-profit United States Green Building Council (USGBC). LEED was among the first systems used to certify buildings as "green." The program identifies a limited number of features as prerequisites—like a non-smoking designation for indoor air quality—that all buildings must have. It additionally provides a much larger list of features that a building *could* integrate. Points are gained in the LEED assessment if a developer integrates bicycle parking, locates a building near transit, or improves heating and cooling systems. LEED points are awarded for using recycled materials and materials that release fewer pollutants into the air. When a certain number of points are accumulated, certification is granted at a basic, silver, gold, or platinum level.

Since its inception, USGBC has created additional rating systems targeted toward different types of buildings: new construction, existing buildings, commercial interiors, core and shell, homes, and schools; there's even LEED certification for neighborhood development. Currently, the LEED certification is used throughout the United States and in more than a hundred countries around the world, including Canada.

At Fit City 1, architects had suggested that we create incentives for the integration of health into the design and construction of built-environment projects. Deborah wondered whether one such incentive could be the creation of a new health-related credit for LEED. Since LEED certification had been in use for several years and was already a familiar tool for building-feature innovation, the creation of a health-related LEED credit seemed like a natural next step—one that had the potential to encourage architects and developers to more routinely integrate features that those of us in the public health field wanted to see in building projects. What we were hoping for included more visible and aesthetically pleasing staircases to encourage daily use; elevators with doors that close more slowly in order to both accommodate those with disabilities and discourage people capable of climbing a few floors from using them; exercise amenities both inside and outside the buildings to promote physical activity; gardening spaces on building grounds or building roofs to promote availability of healthy food, with more porous, less heat-generating non-concrete surfaces; and spaces to support women to continue to breastfeed after their return to work.

Rather than creating one health credit covering every healthy building feature, I thought perhaps we could break down the list and offer more than one health credit. For example, we could create one credit for physical activity, one for urban agriculture, perhaps another one to promote breastfeeding. I met with Deborah again to review my ideas, and also reached out to others I'd met at the Fit City 1 lunch. One of them was Joyce Lee.

At the time, Joyce was the chief architect for the New York

City Mayor's Office of Management and Budget. In that role, she was involved in the budgetary considerations for City of New York building- and construction-related projects. Fortunately for us, Joyce had a strong propensity for innovation, though she naturally had to temper that with consideration of budgetary constraints. When Joyce heard me speak about my desire to create a new LEED credit for health, she was hooked. She pulled me aside after a group meeting of other architects and designers who had given me their business cards at the first Fit City conference. Joyce mentioned that there were a number of New York City government construction and renovation projects that had recently begun design discussions. She suggested picking one of them as a "test subject" for creating a credit. We decided we would start with a credit to promote physical activity. The very next day, she emailed me about a follow-up meeting.

Later, in a large fourteenth-floor conference room at 2 Lafayette Street, down the hall from my office, Joyce showed me the list of new construction and renovation projects, and there it was: the Riverside Health Center, a 1960s Upper West Side building owned by New York's health department. The design process had just started, and Joyce invited me to join the development team.

The LEED green-building rating system would now take into account features related to physical activity, and it would be put into effect for the first time at Riverside. Joyce and I were leading the initiative, and during the remainder of 2006 and into 2007 we met regularly with the Riverside Health Center Project Team, often in the bright, sunlit conference room at the offices of 1100 Architects in Chelsea. The regulars in our not-so-little group included: Ellen Murphy from 1100 Architects; Sally Yap, the health department architect; Zydnia Nazario, the architect who served as the Department of Design and Construction Sustainability point person; and the environmental design firm Atelier Ten, the LEED consultant on the project.

The work was underway, but results weren't going to be achieved overnight. It would take many revisions, and two years of collaboration between Joyce and me and the USGBC head office in Washington, D.C., for the team to write the Innovation Credit for Physical Activity in the manner required for final approval. In the end, the improvements we identified included stair and elevator design features to promote stair use among those who are able, and recreation and exercise space in worksites for use before or after work, and during work breaks and lunch hours. If a design team, like ours, incorporated enough of these features, they would get an extra point toward their LEED certification.

The completed Riverside Health Center was eventually awarded both a New York City Public Design Commission Award for Excellence in Design (2009) and a LEED gold certification. The center is a shining example of the ways in which healthy design features can be integrated into our modern buildings. Although the understated four-story, low-rise institutional building looks like nothing very special from the outside, its new design completely transformed the old, outdated interior and embraced the integration of activity-promoting elements. A second elevator was installed—it's a health center, after all, and not everyone will be capable of taking the stairs—but so was a second staircase, along with signs encouraging its use. One helpfully points out that "When you go up, your blood pressure goes down." And the former cellar was expanded and excavated, making room for, among other things, an employee fitness room.

The work hadn't been fast, or easy, but the result was definitely worth the wait, and it was intriguing to see how progress in one area could have an impact in another. Around the same time that Joyce and I were working on the Innovation Credit for Physical Activity in conjunction with the Riverside renovation, we were also tackling an Urban Agriculture Innovation Credit for an affordable housing project. This credit aimed to get another point for developers and design teams integrating urban agriculture spaces on the roofs or available land of their development.

And I was also tackling the issue of physical activity in schools—or, more to the point, the lack thereof. I was trying desperately to come up with ways to improve physical activity opportunities for our school-aged kids. A lot of parties have a vital interest in what goes on in our cities' schools: the Department of Health, certainly, and the Education Department, the schools themselves, and the School Construction Authority (SCA), which has responsibility for school design, construction, and renovation. If a change was going to be made, I'd need to bring quite a few partners on board.

It was with this in mind—and with thoughts of the Innovation Credit for Physical Activity constantly in my head—that I entered my first meeting with Bruce Barrett, the vice president of Architecture and Engineering at New York City's School Construction Authority. I was initially surprised to find that Bruce is a woman, taller than me, with short gray hair and glasses. Bruce got up, smiled, and shook my hand. She introduced her team members, and Joyce Lee, who had also joined us, introduced herself. Then, we got down to the matter at hand.

I asked Bruce about the possibility of using the LEED building-rating system in the greening of schools in New York. She explained that the SCA had developed its own "Green Guide for Schools," and wasn't interested in adopting a new system. Also, Bruce explained, LEED didn't make sense for use in our public schools, which she thought should have more consistency in their features than was encouraged by a system full of optional points. No doubt responding to my look of discouragement, Bruce rounded out her answer with "But we can see what concepts we can integrate into our own system."

And with that, Bruce became a crucial partner. Together we worked on the integration of the stair use, active recreation, and features promoting walking and bicycle riding to school—modes encompassed in what is called "active transportation"—as new points in the "Green Guide for Schools." We also launched initiatives to ensure that new school construction and school renovation projects would introduce bicycle parking, stair-promoting signage, and even gymatoriums. Taking the place of a traditional auditorium, the gymatorium is a gymnasium convertible to an auditorium, and its presence functionally doubles a school's available physical education and activity space.

I couldn't have hoped for a better outcome—for my own department's goals, or for the children of New York City. Sometimes, all you have to do is ask.

Next Steps: The Active Design Guidelines

In the fall of 2006, with work on the Riverside Health Center and the LEED Innovation Credit for Physical Activity underway but far from completion, it was once again time for Fit City planning. At this point, the goal I was working towards with the conference was engaging as many city departments as possible in the creation and application of a set of principles for supporting active and healthy living that would routinely be incorporated into features in our buildings, streets and neighborhoods, a set of principles that would come to be collectively called Active Design.

I met with Rick Bell at AIANY's Center for Architecture. Rick, speaking at his usual hundred-mile-per-minute speed, would throw out ideas, and I would pick out the ones I thought had potential to promote and enhance the conference and achieve the needed buy-in from key stakeholders. I knew, for example, that I wanted more department commissioners to attend, in order to demonstrate the highest levels of local government support for Active Design principles. Rick mentioned that New York

City's Department of Design and Construction (DDC)—the local equivalent to a Department of Public Works—involved itself in both the building and street aspects of city construction. We toyed with the idea of inviting the commissioner of Design and Construction to attend, but Rick and I both knew we'd run the risk of him sending a staff person. So we added a hook, and asked him to be one of our keynote speakers. He accepted. It turned out to be an important link in the chain that led to the creation of the Active Design Guidelines.

The thinking behind the Active Design Guidelines initiative had three components. First, I wanted to synthesize and gather the most up-to-date evidence regarding the built-environment factors that could promote physical activity and health—particularly to address obesity and diabetes, the two worsening epidemics in New York. Second, I wanted to make that information readily available, in a user-friendly format, to built-environment professionals, including architects, landscape architects, urban designers, urban planners, transportation planners and officials, developers, and others. Third, I wanted to get to a place where these professionals would be *expected* to use the guidelines and routinely integrate health-related factors and considerations in their work. The question, as always, was how to make it all happen.

Fit City 2 took place in May 2007, and things finally started to come together. Confirming the commissioner of the Department of Design and Construction as a keynote speaker was one stroke of luck. The second came when he arrived an hour ahead of his scheduled address and sat in on the other keynote speaker's session. Dr. Craig Zimring, a behavioral psychologist at Georgia Tech's College of Architecture, was talking about the importance of evidence-based design, and he was making some excellent points. Gone are the days, he told the attentive audience, when doctors would treat patients based on their hunches. These days, we expect our medical professionals to treat us based on scientifically supported evidence that the medicine or surgery prescribed has in fact been shown to be effective. We've long since given up the notion of attaching leeches to patients to "bleed" them of whatever ailments they might have. And we now know that there's no point treating a common cold with a course of antibiotics. We've made this progress thanks to decades, even centuries, of research and the evidence that's been accumulated as a result. Why have we not made that leap in other professions? Why do we not expect architects, designers, builders and urban planners to carry out their work based on the evidence of what is effective in addressing societal needs—including tackling modern-day epidemics like obesity and diabetes? Why do we not expect our politicians to enact policies around city and community design and construction based on the evidence of their ability to produce health and other important outcomes? To drive home his point, Craig shared some of that evidence, including the 2001 and 2005 studies by the U.S. Task Force on Community Preventive Services that showed health-conscious design of human-built environments was associated with 35 to 161 percent increases in regular physical activity. When buildings were designed, for example, to encourage stair use instead of elevator use, many people took the stairs (my own observations at Apple stores and AIANY certainly supported this), and we could increase physical activity through stair use by 50 percent. And if people had access to physical activity facilities, even in their workplaces, they would more often use them, and maintain healthier weights as a result. People who live in more walkable communities do indeed walk more.

Craig's keynote was well received by the Fit City 2 audience—which, I was pleased to see, was about twice the size of the inaugural conference's crowd. And it clearly made an impact on the DDC commissioner, too. After the conference, he called to let me

know that he'd support the creation of a set of health-pro[...]
guidelines for city construction.

Buy-in from the DDC was huge. It meant that the City of New York, a large, prominent, influential global city, was now going to create a set of guidelines that it would use in its own street and building design and construction. This would encompass most street construction, which is largely done by the public sector, as well as the design and construction of government buildings which house large numbers of people employed by and served by our governments and government-affiliated institutions (public colleges, libraries, museums, etc.). The potential for population impact was thus very broad.

But now, the truly challenging work began: creating the guidelines. I went back to Lynn and Mary Bassett, Lynn's boss at the health department, and I asked for money. I needed to hire a project coordinator, and I also needed money for academic consultants who could conduct updated literature reviews, identifying and synthesizing the latest available evidence about built-environment supports for health. The initial team meeting with DDC included Craig, Joyce, and me. At that time, we identified others we felt were vital to our working group, and we invited the New York City Departments of City Planning and Transportation to come on board. At our next meeting, Alex Washburn, City Planning's director of Urban Design, showed up, as did Wendy Feuer, an assistant commissioner at the Department of Transportation. Wendy brought in an intern, Hanna Gustaffson, and Alex assigned Skye Duncan, one of his most talented and dedicated designers, to work with Wendy's team on what would become the section of the guidelines related to urban design. Craig suggested inviting Dr. Gayle Nicoll, formerly one of his PhD students and now chair of Architecture at the University of Texas in San Antonio. The health department came through with funding, and I began interviewing candidates for the position of Built Environment Coordinator, reporting to me. Sarah Wolf, a dietician with a master's degree in public health, got the job. Our team was growing fast.

It was finally time to get down to work. Sarah and I wrote the first chapter of the guidelines, which introduced the topic of health and the built environment and its history. We made it a point to highlight the successful lessons from public health and planning in earlier periods. For example, in many of our cities, it was built-environment improvements such as the creation of sanitation systems and clean water, or the introduction of building codes and zoning, that helped us to address the infectious disease epidemics and rampant safety issues of years past. Wendy's team and Skye got to work on the second chapter, on urban design; Dr. Reid Ewing, from the Department of City and Metropolitan Planning at the University of Utah, provided help with the evidence reviews. They identified the evidence for and drafted strategies that would promote walking, biking, and transit use, which often begins and ends with a walk. Their work also focused on ensuring sufficient population density in areas to support "mixed land use," or using available land to support different types of amenities that people could easily walk to. They identified strategies for connecting these uses or amenities with safe and aesthetically pleasing pedestrian and bicycle paths. They identified what could be done with parking and with transit to further promote modes of transportation that would increase physical activity, decrease pollution, and increase safety—in other words, providing better, safer, more pleasant access to transportation choices other than the automobile. Dr. Gayle Nicoll wrote much of the chapter on building design, with assistance from one of Craig's PhD students, Julie Brand Zook. They fleshed out the evidence on factors that would encourage stair use and decrease sedentariness and promote bouts of activity within buildings. Gayle was very familiar with such studies, having done many of the innovative and groundbreaking studies looking at promoting stair use. With Joyce, I also tackled the final chapter, which identified the synergies with other key priorities in New York and elsewhere, including accessibility for those with disabilities and the sustainability of our environment. Joyce and I would integrate the LEED Innovation Credit for Physical Activity into this chapter. And the DDC commissioner had assigned one of his assistant commissioners, Margot Woolley, as well as Victoria Milne, director of Design Services, to assist the team. Victoria, in particular, would play a crucial role by taking on the design and publication of the guidelines document itself, including the layout and graphics, and contracting the needed editorial, production, and printing teams.

Nine months later, we had a completed first draft. I was thrilled to have made it that far, and pleased with the work our team had done, but I dreaded sending the guidelines out for feedback. I was worried that those who opposed the idea could potentially kill it, or, at the very least, dampen enthusiasm straight out of the gate. But I absolutely knew this was a crucial part of the process. If an initiative of this size and complexity is to truly succeed, it needs across-the-board buy-in. Although DDC undertook the design and construction of City buildings, it did so only with the approval of its internal clients, the City departments themselves, whose staff would be working in the buildings. Also, there were a host of other departments that undertook design and construction work separately from DDC and Transportation. For example, the School Construction Authority designed and constructed public schools. The Department of Housing Preservation and Development partnered with private-sector for-profit and non-profit developers to create or expand affordable housing and mixed-income housing. The Department of Parks and Recreation designed and constructed our city parks and playgrounds. The Department of Citywide Administrative Services (DCAS) maintained the buildings, and it could potentially derail the implementation of health-promoting strategies out of concern for the cost or feasibility for building maintenance or security (e.g., strategies like leaving stairwell doors unlocked on all floors, including high-security floors, might be opposed by DCAS for good reason). The Department of Buildings needed to ensure that there were no conflicts between the strategies promoted by our evidence-based studies and the building codes that mandated or allowed what was done in the City's buildings. We needed the wisdom of those who worked in the Department for the Aging to help ensure we were also addressing seniors' issues. The Mayor's Office for People with Disabilities and Office of Sustainability clearly also needed to weigh in to address these issues. And so, I confronted my worries head-on: in order to deal with the opposition, I first needed to know where it might be coming from. Once I knew that, I could turn my attention to addressing concerns and getting any skeptics onside.

In mid 2008, with our draft guidelines document completed and reviewed by the authors, I asked the DDC commissioner to send out an email I'd drafted: this would go to every commissioner of a City agency whose work could be affected by the new guidelines. I asked for their review and feedback, knowing that the commissioners would likely pass the draft on to their assistant commissioners and directors, and in turn some would pass them down to their staff. I wanted to hear any concerns, right down to the staff level if possible. I wanted their suggestions regarding sections that were missing—or, better yet, their drafts of those sections! In the end, we had five City departments involved in co-writing the four chapters, and input from the eight other City departments.

Now, about fifteen months into the process, we had a revised draft that included input and endorsement from thirteen City government agencies, in particular the ones identified above—the departments of Health and Mental Hygiene, Design and

Construction, Planning, Transportation, the Mayor's Offices of Management and Budget, Long-Term Planning and Sustainability, and for People with Disabilities, and the departments for the Aging, Parks and Recreation, Buildings, Housing Preservation and Development, Citywide Administrative Services, and School Construction Authority. The next step was to take the guidelines to several other key stakeholder groups that might also oppose—or support—them. As it had been with the government agencies, the support of these non-governmental stakeholders was vital. These included community, academic, and private-sector stakeholders whose work would be impacted by the guidelines. We needed to include architects, landscape architects, urban designers, and urban planners working in private-sector firms, as well as their clients, like private-sector developers. We needed to know that they could really embrace the guidelines if we were to have any hope of widespread use beyond City construction. Well-known academics in related fields, particularly those who worked and taught in the New York metropolitan area, were invited to share their thoughts. Vocal and well-known advocacy groups for issues like active transportation in the city, such as Transportation Alternatives, were also approached to review the draft guidelines. We certainly wanted these advocacy groups to advocate for use of the guidelines rather than against it!

The team debated how best to ensure that we would get broad inputs from stakeholders. Finally, we decided to invite them to a design workshop. Those who accepted our invitation would be sent the draft of the guidelines, and we'd ask them to show up ready to use those guidelines during the workshop to design streets and buildings. In this way, the workshop would highlight the feasibility and usefulness of the strategies, and it would help us identify things that didn't work.

The workshop was set for January 2009—a year and a half after the meeting that had initiated the creation of the Active Design

Guidelines. Eight or so rectangular tables were set up in the main conference space at the Center for Architecture, and Rick Bell and his AIANY staff were there to help facilitate. Once our guests arrived, we began with a presentation about the guidelines. We then identified the building types and street-scale projects for the design exercise at each table, and let the participants select the projects that best suited their interests. Some people landed themselves at the affordable housing design table. Others went to the design table for regular housing that is bought and sold, or rented, at usual costs driven by the housing market. Others found themselves at a table where design plans were being brainstormed for a worksite building. Some people seated themselves around a project for street design improvements.

At the end of the morning, a whole-group discussion was facilitated, and some consistent themes emerged. We heard that people using the guideline document wanted less text and more pictures. We heard support for the inclusion of case studies at the end of each chapter, particularly the chapters on urban design and building design. We heard that it would be useful to have synergies discussed throughout the document, and not just in the final chapter. Overall, however, people seemed very excited and positive about the initiative. We even heard from some that they couldn't wait to start using the guidelines!

After the workshop, our group reassembled and got down to the task of incorporating all of the excellent feedback we'd received. Over the next year, we trimmed text-dense sections, found more photographs and images, and assembled more case studies. And wherever possible we added discussions of synergies around environmental sustainability and universal accessibility issues. We also worked hard on the final design of the book, using mock layouts and graphics and color schemes. The details were mind-boggling, but it was so satisfying to see all of our hard work coming together.

Christmas came and went, and on December 26, 2009, I was at

my brother's house, a bit north of snowy Edmonton, Alberta. We had just finished our Christmas celebration with a houseful of extended family when an email appeared on my BlackBerry. Our editor, Irene Cheng, had sent along a proof of the final version. Did we want to do one more read? I stared at my phone and tried to figure out what to do. As the lead on the project, I had proofread the document about a hundred times already—so many drafts to arrive, finally, at this one. Did I really need to read it again? I'd corrected all the mistakes on the version I'd read just one week ago, *right?* But what if we'd missed a mistake or two? What if someone had neglected to make one or two of my edits from last week? Reluctantly, I excused myself, went into the room that served as my brother's home office, and closed the door. I turned on the desktop computer and opened the final document. It had come such a long way, and had grown into a much better and more useful piece of work, thanks to all of the input and advice we'd received. At around 11:00 p.m., with just a few more changes noted, I pressed the Send button. I went to bed happy— and slept soundly in the knowledge that two and a half years' worth of work would finally be off to the printer the next day.

A month later, on January 29, 2010, a gathering was held at the AIANY Center for Architecture. In a festive evening event complete with wine, beer, non-alcoholic beverages, and appetizers, the *Active Design Guidelines* was officially launched.

Printed copies of the book were on hand, and e-copies were available to download from the City's website. We monitored visits to the site and found that architects and urban planners from across the world were downloading the document. It appears the New York architects and urban designers who had heard about the guidelines through our emails, workshop, and launch event, or through their colleagues who had received our emails or attended these events, had helped to spread the word far and wide. It was probably helpful as well that many architecture and design firms headquartered in New York also had offices and projects nationally and internationally. At first, this international traffic came from just a few countries, but within months—as word spread— more and more countries downloaded the guidelines. Eventually, we learned that they were being used in more than a hundred countries around the world. The Active Design movement was afoot. As we celebrated our work on the night of our launch, we were hopeful that those who used the guidelines and its strategies would start to design and construct buildings, streets, and neighborhoods—and amenities within them—that would promote the implementation of active transportation, active play, active buildings—and even actively promote healthy food and beverage access—in the world around us.

The Active Design Supplement: Preventing Injuries

It didn't take long for the Active Design Guidelines to have an impact. It was February 2011, and I was happy enough to leave New York's gray, snowy winter behind for San Diego. I smiled as I stepped out of the airport into the warmth of the sunshine to catch a taxi to the Hard Rock Hotel, where the Active Living Research Conference was being held. I was there to represent the Active Design Guidelines team from New York. The conference organizers had invited us to accept the Translating Research to Policy Award. Given out by the Active Living Research Program (ALR), funded by the Robert Wood Johnson Foundation, the award was in its fourth year of recognizing organizations, teams, and projects that best represented the translation of research evidence on the built environment and physical activity into policies for changing our buildings, streets, neighborhoods, and their amenities in the real world. Gayle Nicoll and Joyce Lee would be joining me, but I was preparing to make a presentation about our project as a part of accepting the award at the conference.

The next day, as our team was announced at the award ceremony, I made my way to the stage, and Dr. Jim Sallis, director of the ALR program, came up to shake my hand. Jim waved his arms up and down, indicating to the audience that they should stand up and participate in his favorite conference invention: active applause. Jim reminded those who had missed his opening remarks that active applause—standing up to offer congratulations after every presentation—was the practice at ALR events. It was good for the audience to be less sedentary, and it made the presenter feel good too!

I made a presentation about the Active Design Guidelines, and afterwards, during the break, I was approached by David Sleet, a senior staff member at the U.S. Centers for Disease Control and Prevention, in the National Center for Injury Prevention. He thought it would be great if we could create something similar to the Active Design Guidelines for preventing injuries, both intentional (such as those related to crime) and unintentional (such as those related to motor vehicle crashes). Did I have any thoughts? He already had a contract with the Society for Public Health Education (SOPHE) and funding he could provide for such a project. If I was interested, he would find SOPHE executive director Elaine Auld, who was also attending the conference, and introduce us.

I was, of course, enthusiastic. I told David I'd love to see if we could identify the Active Design Guideline strategies that would synergistically reduce injuries, regardless of their cause. Those strategies would give communities and cities a double bang for every dollar spent implementing them. Injuries are the leading cause of death in North America for those under the age of forty-five, and are also a leading killer globally, particularly injuries related to motor vehicles. And physical inactivity is a leading risk factor for preventable non-communicable diseases, which are now the leading causes of death—period—around the world.

Being able to prevent both by using the same strategies would be incredibly valuable, not to mention cost- and resource-efficient.

And that is how I came to meet Elaine Auld, and, through her, Andrea Gielen, director of the Center for Injury Research and Policy at Johns Hopkins University's Bloomberg School of Public Health. Elaine suggested I meet with her and Andrea for lunch the next day at the hotel's café. As we sat at a pine table, eating our to-go meals, we kicked around ideas. Elaine could funnel some of the CDC funding to Andrea's team for the literature reviews specifically focusing on the impacts that the Active Design Guidelines would be expected to have on injuries. And I would use my team to coordinate the project, bringing on board key New York City department stakeholders from Health, Transportation, Buildings, and Parks. Additional community and advocacy groups would also be engaged. The perspectives of these policy-makers in key departments whose practices impacted safety would be integral to the document's creation, as well as to ensure buy-in and feasible implementation. As the evidence for safety was reviewed by Andrea's group at Johns Hopkins, including Keshia Pollack and Maryanne Bailey, we were able to determine that many evidence-based strategies to support physical activity—like more visible and well-lit stairs—also promoted safety. And strategies to prevent injury among pedestrians and cyclists would also serve to promote walking and cycling. Streetlights to prevent crime, better street crossings to prevent pedestrian–motor vehicle collisions—the strategies to promote physical activity and safety overlapped to a great extent.

In 2012, after multiple rounds of reviews, the document *Active Design Supplement: Promoting Safety* was published in both a hardcopy format and as a downloadable e-copy hosted by the Johns Hopkins Center for Injury Research and Policy on its website.

Clearly, the movement was picking up momentum.

5 | FIRST STEPS

THE MOVEMENT IN ACTION

The secret of change is to focus all of your energy, not on fighting the old, but on building the new.

—SOCRATES

Whatever good things we build end up building us.

—JIM ROHN

YOU COULD BE forgiven for thinking that my entire time with the New York City Department of Health and Mental Hygiene was spent on the Active Design Guidelines and Fit City conferences! They were both big aspects of the work to make progress on, and vital stepping-stones for, the work I wanted to do in terms of health and the built environment. And the relationships I made working on these projects were central to so much of the good work that came out of them. Without Fit City, there would have been no Active Design Guidelines, and without the Active Design Guidelines, I'm not sure how successful I would have been with some of the other initiatives I was so eager to get off the ground. But as time-consuming and exhausting as the work on conferences and guidelines was, it didn't happen in a vacuum. As the Active Design movement gained momentum, my colleagues and I had many opportunities to put our ideas into action, both in New York and farther afield.

"The Little Sign That Could"

When I arrived in New York from Atlanta, with my CDC experiences in West Virginia fresh in my mind, I was eager to get one particular initiative off the ground: the development of a sign that would encourage people to take the stairs. Simple, right?

Not exactly. Flash-forward to the Fit City 3 conference in May 2008 (and note the date: *two years* after I started my work in New York). I'm watching from the front row, sitting among roughly three hundred other audience members in the darkened room. Dr. Thomas Frieden, commissioner of the New York City Department of Health, and Rick Bell, executive director of the New York chapter of the American Institute of Architects, are standing at the front of the room, under bright lights that illuminate a large sign on a stand. The sign—three feet by two feet—features a white stick figure climbing a white staircase pitched against a bright, lime-green background. Above the figure, in white, are the words "Burn Calories, Not Electricity." Below the figure, also in white, is "Take the Stairs."

It was such a simple message, presented in such a simple way. And yet, I knew only too well how much hard work it had taken to get to this day. Two years of cooperation with the Department of Health and Mental Hygiene's assistant commissioner of Communications, Geoffrey Cowley, and the Department of Design and Construction's design services team led by Victoria Milne. Two years of working toward sign-off and endorsement from multiple partners, including Mayor Bloomberg's GreeNYC Office (the public campaigns side of the Mayor's Office of Long-Term Planning and Sustainability), AIANY, and the Real Estate Board of New York, the city's most powerful lobby group. Two years of meetings and memos and late nights and compromises geared toward the creation of a sign that was more than just something I dreamed up on my own, one that featured the logos of the key partners who supported the initiative. Yes, *two years* for this "simple" sign to be finalized and released.

Little did I know when we started working on this sign that it would garner enough attention to be used not only in New York but in Oregon, in California, in Atlanta (at the offices of the National Center for Environmental Health at the U.S. CDC), elsewhere in the United States, and even as far away as London, England, and at the University of Alberta in Canada.

In many ways, it was "the little sign that could," a symbol for me—and other like-minded people—of what the Active Design movement could accomplish with creative thinking, dedication, and cooperation. It was, no doubt, a step in the right direction. We were off and climbing.

Testing . . . Testing . . .

I first met Nancy Biberman, founder and executive director of the Women's Housing and Economic Development Corporation (WHEDco), in 2008 not long after the "Take the Stairs" sign had been unveiled. When our paths crossed, I was busy looking for places to integrate and test the stair-prompt sign, the ideas we were working into the Active Design Guidelines, and the LEED Innovation Credit for Physical Activity. Nancy was putting the finishing touches on her second affordable housing development, Intervale Green, which was striving to improve both quality and sustainability in affordable housing developments.

Intervale Green, located in the Bronx, was a direct result of Mayor Bloomberg's goal to build or preserve 165,000 affordable housing units during his tenure. According to the Guide for Community Preventive Services, tenant-based rental-assistance programs that provide low-income families with more housing options had been shown to improve health-related outcomes. Additionally, where there are health disparities and inequities resulting from the built environment, improving the designs and amenities in and around affordable housing developments could assist families with restricted incomes who could not otherwise afford some of the health-promoting amenities or programs that others of us might take for granted (e.g., gym membership, children's sports programs). Even access to safe and convenient transportation modes that are not car-dependent could be a very important measure to improve health equity. There are studies showing, for example, that households living in completely car-dependent neighborhoods are sometimes required to spend roughly 25 percent of their household income on transportation, while households living in neighborhoods with options to walk, bicycle, or take transit might spend only 9 percent. For those with limited incomes, being able to get by without a car could mean having money for healthier food and for active recreation programs for their children. If certain jobs and needed services require a car to get there, it could also prevent those who cannot afford a car to have less access to such jobs and services.

In many ways, Intervale Green exemplified New York's new approach to affordable housing developments. In this model, the building and running of the development was left to private-sector developers—some for-profit, others non-profit like WHEDco—who would use funding and incentives provided by federal, state, and local governments to subsidize construction and maintenance. Frequently, middle-income and even market-rate apartments for purchase might be included as part of the building's offerings and used to help offset the costs of not only construction, but maintenance over time, of the affordable or subsidized units.

Trained as a lawyer, Nancy had founded WHEDco in 1992 to help low-income women and their children, many from the homeless shelter system, with housing, education, and economic development opportunities. Headquartered in the South Bronx, on the tenth floor of their first affordable housing development, Urban Horizons, WHEDco has since developed three affordable housing developments in the neighborhood.

At our first meeting, Nancy and I discussed opportunities for collaboration. Yes, she was interested in putting up our stair-prompt signs in both Urban Horizons and Intervale Green. And yes, she was interested in being a site for a study evaluating the impact of those signs on stair use and physical activity. So far, so good. And then it got even better. While it was too late to change Intervale Green's design, Nancy was willing to explore the possibility of simple and inexpensive interventions.

That first discussion was fruitful in several ways. It helped to solidify the importance of Nancy's idea to create Intervale Green's rooftop garden, where interested residents enjoy access to both fresh produce and physical activity. It led to "painting days," approximately once a year, to create new mural art on the walls of the building's stairwell, one floor at a time. And it led to WHEDco's participation as one of three sites where the impact of our stair-prompt signs was evaluated.

That study took me back to my time in West Virginia. It was definitely a "boots on the ground" operation. Vicky Grimshaw from my staff, and Ashley Perry, our Master of Public Health graduate intern, joined me to hit the pavement—or, in Ashley's case, the bench. Perched on a bench in the Urban Horizons lobby, Ashley tried to be inconspicuous as she counted the number of people taking the stairs and the number of people taking the elevators, and took note of the direction in which they were traveling. Ashley conducted these counts at the WHEDco building in the South Bronx before the stair-prompt signs went up. And she would count them again immediately after the signs went up, then several weeks later, and then, finally, nine months later.

Vicky and Ashley would also travel to the Riverside Health Center to repeat the exercise. One of them would stand near the elevator and observe people as they traveled either up from the lobby or down to the basement, where food safety and other courses were taught. The other would stand in the stairwell, observing those who entered and the direction in which they moved.

When Ashley was not in the field, she'd be at her desk, diligently entering her data. We, in turn, would use that data to calculate rates of stair use versus elevator use both before and after the installation of the stair-prompt signs; rates of stair climbing versus elevator use going up; and rates of stair descent versus elevator use going down. In a paper we co-authored for the *American Journal of Preventive Medicine,* we showed that the placement of the "Burn Calories, Not Electricity. Take the Stairs!" sign next to elevator call buttons and outside stairwells increased stair use immediately after posting, increased stair climbing as well as stair descent, and increased stair use significantly even nine months after placement.

Over the year or so that Ashley was with our team, she worked in the field many times. In addition to helping us collect data for the stair vs. elevator use evaluation studies, she also helped us assess what buildings did with the stair-prompt signs once they received the orders for them. We started with a list of 118 buildings whose managers or owners had called New York City's 311 information line and ordered the stair-prompt signs between May and September of 2008, after the launch at our Fit City 3 conference. From there we narrowed it down to 58 buildings in Manhattan, Brooklyn, and the Bronx. These boroughs were targeted because they housed three of the health department's highest-priority areas in terms of health needs: East and Central Harlem in Manhattan, the South Bronx, and North and Central Brooklyn. Ashley's job was to report on whether those who had ordered the stair-prompt signs were using them, and where they were placing them.

In the spring of 2009, Ashley would take the subway to her "neighborhood of the day." Dressed in comfortable walking shoes and business-casual khakis—a public health worker's field uniform if ever there was one—she would walk to the buildings on her list. Some were locked and inaccessible. At others she would flash her New York City Department of Health and Mental Hygiene badge and then wait while the doorman or guard checked to see if she could enter. If she wasn't sent away, she'd wait patiently until she was told to go ahead, or until someone came to escort her around. In the end, Ashley assessed twenty-four buildings and was able to write a report showing that about half of those had posted the stair-prompt signs. She learned that buildings with stair access from the lobby and/or other floors were more likely to have posted the stair-prompt signs than those that had no stair access or restricted access. It seemed that good access to stairs was an important complementary measure for stair-prompt posting.

That last bit of information led to further action. In 2010, after publication of the *Active Design Guidelines*, I hired a staff member specifically to help me help those building owners and managers. Johnny Adamic was in his late twenties, a young man from Wisconsin who would bound up eight flights of stairs every morning on his way to our office—he definitely practiced what he preached when it came to stair use and physical activity. He was the perfect person to make building owners and managers more aware of the free stair-promoting signs, and to help them post them correctly. Johnny had a master's degree in a field completely unrelated to health, or even to the built environment, but he had worked for a year between his undergraduate and graduate degrees selling hospital building equipment, like handrails. I knew his enthusiastic attitude would be what we needed to help us implement our stair-prompt strategy successfully. Johnny would get the building managers and operators he worked with to order the best type of signage—styrene rather than paper—to stay up permanently next to the elevators and outside stairwells. He would create a package of materials to send out with the signs that were ordered, like good adhesives to both post the signs and keep them up on the walls. And, never one to let an opportunity go to waste, Johnny would also pass along a copy of the *Active Design Guidelines* and encourage those he visited to integrate other strategies if possible.

From 2008 through the remainder of the Bloomberg administration, nearly forty thousand stair-prompt signs were distributed to over a thousand buildings in New York City.

The Green Codes Report: Planning for Healthy Growth

In 2007—when I was in the midst of my work on the LEED credit, the Riverside Health Center, and the stair-prompt sign—New York City launched PlaNYC 2030. In anticipation of the population growth projected for the city, from 8.2 million residents to an anticipated 9 million by 2030, the Mayor's Office of Long-Term Planning and Sustainability was calling for a serious discussion. How would this population growth be managed? New York was already a crowded and congested city. When I first arrived in New York, traffic jams were a constant, day or night, weekday or weeknight. The streets of Manhattan, particularly in places like Times Square, were overcrowded with people crammed onto not-wide-enough sidewalks. Housing was expensive and already increasingly unaffordable to many. Public parks that were present were already very well used by an increasing number of people living here. Many of the parks that were available, like Central Park in Manhattan and Prospect Park in Brooklyn, were built in the 1800s. More parks for this growing population were sorely needed. Now we needed to house, move, and provide healthy, open, active spaces for another nearly one million new people. We knew that, if nothing else, we needed to ensure that the additional million or so people didn't make all of the city's challenges even worse.

In a series of meetings with key infrastructure agencies, the Mayor's Office asked some important questions: How could the government ensure that the city would remain environmentally sustainable, and that quality of life would be maintained— or even improved—for its residents? How could it ensure that the growth of the city would not be accompanied by even worse traffic congestion, air pollution, and overcrowding or loss of available and accessible recreational spaces? Goals and objectives were set. Supports for walking, cycling, and public transit as viable and desirable modes of transportation was a key proposal. Having every New York City resident live within a ten-minute walk of a park or playground was another. Where large parks might be missing or impossible to add, small pocket parks, including pedestrian plazas, would be used. I followed the discussions with interest. If ideas like this came to fruition, there would be sweeping changes indeed. The objectives also introduced key opportunities to promote and protect health, and I knew the next version of PlaNYC would need to include health outcomes explicitly.

Following the launch of PlaNYC 2030 as New York City's master plan for growth, policies were enacted to help ensure its goals were met. In 2009, I was presented with an opportunity to take part in the policy-making process when Laurie Kerr, senior adviser in the Office of Long-Term Planning and Sustainability, got in touch. Laurie and I had known each other for a few years; in fact, it was during a working session around a joint panel presentation for the national conference of the American Institute of Architects in 2007 that she and I had come up with a phrase— "diseases of energy"—to describe the non-communicable diseases whose risk factors of physical inactivity and unhealthy diets were linked to the overconsumption of external energy sources and an underutilization of the energy within our own bodies. Laurie told me that a task force was being formed with Urban Green, the New York City chapter of the U.S. Green Building Council. The goal of the task force was to undertake the work, as described in earlier sections of this book, to "green" the city's design and construction codes from building right on down to plumbing. Laurie wanted the Green Codes Task Force to include a Health and Physical Activity Technical Committee. Would I be willing to serve as co-chair?

We'd come a long way since 2006. It had been only three years since my work in New York had begun, and now health and physical activity considerations were being integrated into numerous city policies and processes—even those that, on the surface, seemed to have nothing to do with "health." And I was being invited to participate in initiatives, such as this one, that once would have had no health representation or consideration. I said yes, of course, I'd be pleased to accept.

We got down to work immediately. The committee, like the other eight technical committees formed, would have only a few months to brainstorm and then finalize a set of recommendations that would green New York City's construction codes and, in our case, simultaneously promote physical activity and health. We knew we needed the best people to help, and so we invited William Stein, a private-sector architect with the firm Dattner Architects, to co-chair. Bill was, after all, the lead architect on a project that won an affordable design competition, a project his team called Via Verde, or the Green Way (see chapter 6 for more on this project). I knew Bill, and Bill was familiar with our work on integrating physical activity and health into building, site, and community design. Even before the time of our Green Codes committee, Bill had already agreed that his team would use the Active Design Guidelines and integrate the LEED

Innovation Credit for Physical Activity into Via Verde. We filled out the committee with a combination of senior staff from city departments, including Planning and Buildings, and representatives from private-sector architecture and engineering firms.

The day of our first committee meeting arrived. I had invited Dr. Gayle Nicoll, who had worked with us in drafting the Active Design Guidelines, to present potential opportunities for the committee members to consider: opportunities that could be incorporated through allowances in the international building codes; that were being used in other jurisdictions; and that were being shown by health and building research to be important but not currently implemented in real-world buildings.

Via conference call from San Antonio, Texas, Gayle presented research on buildings and physical activity, particularly around the facilitation and encouragement of stair use. We heard how visibility of the stairs from the building entrance appeared to be a critical element. We heard how aesthetic elements like music and art, along with design considerations like wider staircases, had been shown to increase stair use. We heard how stair-prompt signage—such as the "Burn Calories, Not Electricity" sign that had been created in New York City the year prior—showed strong evidence of successfully getting people to be more active in their day-to-day lives. Gayle then proceeded to review several pieces of new technology that were now permitted by international building codes. Technologies like magnetic "hold-opens" that could keep stair doors open most of the time, but would demagnetize when a fire alarm rang, allowing the doors to close, such as the one that the American Institute of Architects New York Chapter was already using in their Center for Architecture to promote visibility and use of their main fire stairs. There was also new glass that could withstand fires for an extended period of time without exploding, unlike previous types of glass that couldn't be used to cover large areas of fire-stair doors and walls. We heard how these technologies were now being used, or at least were allowed, in other jurisdictions. For example, in Kentucky's building code, magnetic hold-opens were allowed for use to keep stairwell doors— even fire doors—open, and the stairs more visible.

· The architects on the committee were well aware of all the items *not* permitted by New York City codes, including magnetic hold-opens. And from our individual daily experiences, many of us also knew that stair use in New York could be challenging. Staircases were often relegated to the back corners of buildings. Frequently, the doors to access the stairs were locked. If they did happen to be open, it was not uncommon to find the stairs poorly lit, and painted in a drab gray, if at all. And with our stair-prompt initiative still in its infancy, signage encouraging stair use was hard to find. I also knew that many people were frustrated by the lack of stair access. After the new stair-prompt sign was launched at Fit City 3 and reported in the press, the number one complaint that New Yorkers raised in their comments was lack of stair access; this was brought up in between 20 and 25 percent of all the comments made about the announcement. Many New Yorkers said they *wanted* to use the stairs in the buildings where they worked and lived, but they found it difficult—or even impossible—to do so. I shared this information with the members of my Green Codes Task Force Health and Physical Activity Technical Committee.

In February 2010, one month after the release of the *Active Design Guidelines*, the Green Codes Task Force Report was published and announced at an evening event at City Hall. The room buzzed with excitement as men and women in suits greeted and congratulated each other on a job well done. It was clear that the hundred-plus invitation-only attendees were thrilled, anticipating that the recommendations would become the basis for the next steps to a greener—and also healthier—city. I could see members of my committee scattered here and there across the large second-floor room, a room you entered after ascending the beautiful curved staircase that greeted you in the center of the City Hall lobby right in front of the building's main entrance. Ah—the buildings from the old days, where the staircase was an integral part of the grand entrance!

The staircase, as it turned out, was a major element in our recommendations for environmentally friendly improvements to building and zoning codes. The committee recommended that stair access and stair-use prompts be mandated in all buildings. Access, after all, is critical in terms of supporting a person's choice to take the stairs. Certain buildings were exempt—psychiatric hospitals, for instance, where safety considerations were a very real concern—but for others, the recommendations were clear: the use of stair-promoting features such as width, aesthetic elements (art and music), and improved visibility (through, for example, the use of fire-rated glass) should be encouraged through the creation of zoning incentives. Zoning could allow developers and building owners to widen the stairs if it didn't count the stair floor area toward the maximum floor area allowed for particular buildings and building types. Zoning could even offer additional floor area bonuses—for example, the allowance of an extra floor to be added to a building—if the building's stairwells met certain criteria.

The committee also recommended that magnetic stair hold-open devices be permitted. If international building codes—and other U.S. state codes, like Kentucky's—could allow them, why not New York City building codes? This measure had seemed simple enough to recommend, but if the stair-prompt sign approval process had taught me anything, it was that sometimes "simple" could be pretty complicated. This time, the complications came courtesy of the Fire Department of New York (FDNY). As we tried to take the next steps with the Green Codes Task Force Report—turning recommendations into actual building code changes—we had to work hard to address the FDNY's very legitimate concerns about public safety.

Working with the deputy chief of the FDNY and his staff, Laurie Kerr, Keith Wen (director of codes at the Department of Buildings), and I learned that magnetic hold-opens had been prohibited in New York primarily because of the number of very tall high-rise buildings in the city. In buildings like these, open stairway doors on every floor could create a vacuum effect, sucking flames into the stairwell in the event of a fire.

A meeting—then two, then three before we lost count—took place at the Fire Department's headquarters. With the Brooklyn skyline as a dramatic backdrop, we talked the issue through. We listened to the FDNY's concerns, and they listened to us. The vacuum effect was certainly something that needed to be taken into account, but I pointed out that the department's own report from the 1993 World Trade Center bombings had found that a lack of familiarity with the stairs—from location to layout—was also a major reason for delays in escape from the building. Thus, improving stair visibility and encouraging regular daily stair use by building occupants could also help with safety in the event of an emergency.

It took a bit of time, but we hammered out an agreement. Yes, we could safely allow magnetic hold-open devices to be used, but only on three floors of any given building. The compartmentalizing would negate the vacuum effect. The Green Codes Report recommendations for routine stair access and for use of stair-prompt signs would also help us address the issue of familiarity with stairs. Working together, we were able to balance fire safety precautions with the promotion of regular physical activity for building occupants.

As we sat in that room at FDNY headquarters, it was clear that the many months of working together—and meeting weekly—had created a bond between Laurie, Keith, and me. I was so grateful for these allies who were fighting with me to ensure that physical activity and health choices were available to all building users. Our teamwork paid off in June 2013 when Mayor Michael Bloomberg signed an executive order for Active Design, supported by the Department of Citywide Administrative Services, the Department of Housing Preservation and Development, the Department of Design and Construction, and the Department of Transportation. Moving forward, City agencies would be required to review the design of all City-owned or City-involved construction and major renovation projects to assess opportunities to implement Active Design Guideline elements into buildings and streets. The order also required that agencies assess opportunities to promote the use of stairways, and train design and construction personnel in the use of the Active Design Guidelines.

In 2014, the City took further steps, passing new legislation that allowed magnetic hold-open devices for stairwell doors to be used on up to three floors of a building within New York City's updated greener—and healthier—building codes. With Laurie's support, we also passed legislation to update the plumbing codes in a variety of ways. Among improvements for both health and the environment were requirements that improved tap water infrastructure for drinking water in buildings. Now, not only do new buildings in New York City need to provide drinking water fountains, but those fountains must also be accompanied by water bottle refilling stations. This measure to promote tap water consumption was a win on two fronts: it greens the city *and* it promotes healthier beverage consumption.

Mission accomplished—or, at the very least, firmly underway.

6 | BUILDING MOMENTUM

VIA VERDE, ARBOR HOUSE, AND THE AFFORDABLE HOUSING STUDY

WALKING DOWN BROOK AVENUE in the South Bronx, it's hard not to notice Via Verde. First of all, the structure is not one building but several buildings, of different heights and different shapes. It was constructed that way so the development would fit into an oddly shaped, roughly triangular plot that the City of New York had allocated to a new mixed-income affordable housing development. There are middle-income units that can be purchased, and there are also rental units for those whose incomes are too low to be able to afford to buy. Via Verde was the winner of a design competition held by the City of New York, in partnership with non-governmental organizations like the New York chapter of the American Institute of Architects (AIANY), to improve the design of affordable housing in the city.

Via Verde translates from Spanish as "the Green Way." It's a name that can mean so many things: a green light signifying permission to move forward, environmentally friendly, exposure to the greenery of nature, the opportunity of having green space. Via Verde is all of that and more. Much like Intervale Green, it's a development whose very existence can teach New York, and the world, a lesson. It's a bricks-and-mortar testament to the fact that affordable housing developments (like market-rate housing buildings) can be innovative, environmentally friendly, and health-conscious. And it's one of the first places where I got to see the Active Design ideas in action.

Green Pioneer: Via Verde

My involvement with Via Verde began at yet another AIANY event—this time, a presentation by the four finalists in the New Housing New York Legacy Competition. Sponsored by AIANY, the New York City Department of Housing Preservation and Development (HPD), the New York State Energy Research and Development Authority, and the Enterprise Foundation, the competition had at its heart an admirable goal: to set a new standard for affordable housing by integrating design excellence, sustainability, and the promotion of healthy living. The prize was a triangular lot in the economically disadvantaged South Bronx. I watched, fascinated, as the finalists made their presentations. When the question-and-answer period wrapped up and the lights came on, I made my way over to introduce myself to each of the presenting teams. My hope was that, together, we could concurrently address our modern-day epidemics and issues of health disparities. It was during these introductions that I met Bill Stein, whose team was the eventual winner of the competition. (Bill and I would work together in 2009 on the Green Codes Task Force Health and Physical Activity Technical Committee.) His team's innovative design proposed a twenty-story tower, a mid-rise building, and townhouses, all situated around a central courtyard, part of which would be made up of green spaces on building roofs—Via Verde.

We met many times over the years in which the Via Verde design and construction plans were being developed and finalized. The goal, from the outset, was to integrate strategies from the Active Design Guidelines and the LEED Innovation Credit for Physical

Activity into this new community. We sat around a large conference room table in the offices of Dattner Architects on Fifty-
Seventh Street, near Carnegie Hall, studying a miniature white
plaster model of the design. We discussed stair placement and
what design elements (lighting? color?) might affordably and
feasibly be integrated to increase stair visibility and make the
stairs more pleasant to use. We discussed play areas for children
and activity areas for adults. With the Riverside Health Center
having recently achieved the LEED Innovation Credit for Physical
Activity as a health and worksite building, we wanted Via Verde to
demonstrate that housing—even affordable housing—could
also make the grade. If the winner of a competition for innovation in housing couldn't do it, then what hope would we have for
other housing projects?

Bill and his team, along with Bright Power—leaders in energy
efficiency, solar power, and sustainability—and Grimshaw Architects, a collaborating firm, would bring our discussions back to
their clients, developer Jonathan Rose Companies and building
manager Phipps Houses. We would hear about cost constraints,
concerns about potential liability issues, and worries about security of the spaces. For example, many previous affordable housing
developments were built as social housing for the poor, rather
than as mixed-income housing developments where people of
different socio-economic means might live nearby to each other
such as at Via Verde. Often the social housing of the past would
be poorly maintained since maintenance costs would accumulate over time and yet could not be offset by rent or condo fee
increases. In old social housing, poor maintenance often led to
poor lighting and poor visibility in the stairwells, making them
dangerous spaces with a high potential for crime. Over the
space of a few years, we would work through many of these
issues together.

In the end, Via Verde exceeded all of our expectations. There were so many things to like there. Of the 221 units available, 150 were designated to be rented to households earning between 30 and 90 percent of the median income for the area. The remaining units could be purchased by those whose incomes exceeded these restrictions for the rental units. A large City-owned sports field is located just to the south, easily accessible to Via Verde's residents, and the building itself includes a rooftop state-of-the-art fitness facility that costs less than twenty dollars a year for residents to join. The step-up design of the tower—which starts as a low-rise at the south end before climbing to its full height at the north end—allows maximum access to natural light for both the apartments and the rooftops, which are all green. Evergreen trees, fruit trees, and raised vegetable and garden beds can all be found, adding up to forty thousand square feet of green roof space.

Via Verde also uses simple design innovations to encourage physical activity. Stairways are brightly colored, lit by natural light, and clearly visible from building entries through fire-rated glass doors. Most of the green roofs are usable spaces, with gardening spaces spread throughout, and the courtyard includes a playground and plenty of places for children and adults alike to enjoy being outdoors. To further promote health and well-being, a community medical clinic occupies a ground-floor retail space. Is it any wonder Via Verde received the LEED Innovation Credit for Physical Activity?

We'd set out to prove that affordable housing could also be healthy housing, and we'd gotten the job done. That was satisfying in and of itself. But what made the achievement all the more enjoyable was hearing feedback from the development's residents. An article written for the Robert Wood Johnson Foundation, sponsors of the Active Living Research Program, mentions Raquel Lizardi and her garden club members, who "brave the New York City cold to tend their community's apple trees." Lizardi told the interviewer that she'd lost thirty pounds since moving in. "'I use the gym regularly, but more important, this is not like living in a normal building in Harlem or the Bronx. Here, you don't feel the stress of coming into a dirty building or fearing crime.'"

Via Verde was definitely a win for the Active Design movement, and for affordable housing, but it wasn't an outlier. Despite rumors to the contrary, this wasn't some charmed showpiece, willed into existence only through the support of contest sponsors and a motivated municipal government. No—Via Verde was a leader, a development whose owner, management team, and design team saw where things could be headed and jumped on board early. Others, though, were right there with them.

Arbor House: A Pie-in-the-Sky Idea

It's May 2012 and I'm in the middle of a housing tour arranged as part of the annual Fit City conference. I should be paying attention to what's going on around me, but instead, I'm fixated on the small package in my hands. It's full of baby bok choy, harvested and bagged that same morning. "Sky Vegetables," says the label, with the tag line "Good for you—good for the planet." Another logo, above the package's barcode, reads "Pride of New York."

The Sky Vegetables venture is aptly named. The epitome of locally grown, the vegetables produced here are literally grown in the sky, on a high-rise rooftop in the heart of New York City. When farm manager Kate Ahearn handed me her business card—along with the bok choy—I couldn't help but marvel at the address: 1071 Tinton Avenue, Bronx, New York. The *rooftop* of 1071 Tinton Avenue, to be exact. It was a pie-in-the-sky idea that had taken shape and become a reality, this farm on the rooftop of Arbor House, an affordable housing building in the South Bronx.

Stifling the desire to nibble on the bok choy right then and there, I tuck the package in my backpack and refocus my attention on Kate and her staff, who are giving us the low-down on their work. The day before, twenty or so people had signed up for this outing during registration. Fit City, now in its seventh year, was beginning to attract an international crowd as well as a local one, and since 2010 we had been offering site tours and field visits for interested attendees. The idea was to offer a firsthand look at some of the points of interest that our slides had already presented two-dimensionally. We had a varied group today, some from architecture firms around the city, some from City departments, some hospital and health care staff, and even some guests from London in the U.K.

Arbor House is impressive. At the entrance, we'd noted the sign designating it as a non-smoking building. This offers a benefit to residents, who don't have to deal with the second-hand smoke that would inevitably seep across apartments, and also to the building owner, since smoke creates higher maintenance and insurance costs. We'd seen the building's stairs—walls decorated with stenciled art, risers decked out in colorful paint, and the stairwell humming with music. And we'd checked out the fitness room and outdoor exercise equipment (stationary bike or elliptical, anyone?); some of us had even climbed on to give them a try. Finally, we'd made our way to Sky Vegetables, the hydroponic farm on the rooftop, where Kate Ahearn had proudly handed out samples of her work.

Sunlight pours in through the glass of the beautiful, extensive greenhouse, illuminating row upon row of green vegetables. In addition to the baby bok choy, there's green leaf lettuce, Boston lettuce, and kale. There's a section dedicated to herbs, and new plants being tended in smaller trays. There are rainwater capture bins that help to make the operation even more environmentally friendly.

"Why a hydroponic farm rather than a soil-based farm?" a middle-aged woman with reddish-brown hair and a British accent asks.

It's an interesting question, I think, because hydroponic farms—which employ water and mineral nutrient solutions—are more complex than soil-based farming and must be managed and run by professional staff trained in hydroponic techniques.

Les Bluestone, the owner of Arbor House, makes the point that hydroponic farming "grows a whole lot more food for any farming area you have available." Kate and her staff chime in: hydroponic farms also need less water and fewer pesticides than traditional farms, since there are often fewer pests and weeds to deal with.

"Wow," someone murmurs aloud.

Yes, I think to myself. *Wow, indeed.*

I was introduced to Arbor House fairly early in my tenure with the Department of Health and Mental Hygiene. I was still learning on the job, but I'd figured one thing out for sure: the creation of something extraordinary does not happen without vision, way-above-average efforts, and innovative partnerships. Arbor House was no exception. It came to fruition through the shared vision of an affordable housing developer, Les Bluestone, who believed he could make a difference in the lives of those he housed even as he made a profit; a public health physician (me!) who believed public health departments could return to their roots of healthy community planning and building to mitigate current-day epidemics; and Joyce Lee, chief architect for the Mayor's Office of Management and Budget, who wanted to use her position to help society solve all sorts of thorny issues, from environmental destruction to public health concerns. Buoyed by the successes of such early pilot projects as Intervale Green and Via Verde, the Department of City Planning would also pitch in by removing some of the obstacles these encountered in using their rooftops for needed amenities, from food production to exercise spaces. City Planning would eventually introduce policies to make it easier to build green roofs, freeing up what amounts to acres and acres of unused and underused real estate in one of the world's busiest cities. In the beginning, though, we had no idea where we'd end up. We just knew that opportunity was knocking, and we wanted to answer the door.

The South Bronx contains some of the poorest neighborhoods in both New York City and in the United States as a whole, with median annual household incomes of under $9,000. (In contrast, a twenty-minute ride on New York City's subway system will take you to the Upper East Side, which has some of the wealthiest households.) And affordable housing, among real estate developments, has some of the tightest margins for cost flexibility. In order to keep rental costs low, all attempts are made to also keep the costs of construction and maintenance as low as possible. Therefore, unlike market rate rental or purchased housing that can raise its prices if construction and maintenance costs run over, there is less room for dealing with increased costs and budgets in affordable housing.

Arbor House was already a work in progress when the Bloomberg administration made its commitment to building or preserving 165,000 units of affordable housing, keeping in mind PlaNYC 2030, with its predictions of significant population growth for the city. Ever striving for efficiency, the Bloomberg administration figured that if they were going to be creating housing, they should be creating it in a way that would help solve some of our many problems. Environmental concerns were high on that list, so new housing, like other new construction or renovation projects, needed to be green, particularly if the City was involved in the building's creation, development, or renovation. Health concerns, too—those ever-higher rates of obesity and its related consequences—were a priority. I knew that a need for more housing presented a unique opportunity to address some of our key health challenges.

It was in this context that I had come to know Arbor House's owner. Soon after one of our first Fit City conferences, as we worked on the LEED Innovation Credit for Physical Activity with the design teams for the Riverside Health Center and for Via Verde, Joyce Lee and I also met with Les Bluestone of the Blue Sea Development Company and shared some ideas. Les wasn't at all deterred by the fact that Arbor House—known at the time as Forest House—was already in the late stages of architectural design; he simply asked his architect to take another look and see what could be done. At our second meeting, perhaps a month or two later, Les proudly presented us with a revised design showing that he had moved his main entrance to a different side of the building so it would open onto a lobby where the stairs were located, rather than to the elevator area. "So, this should help to promote more stair use, right?" he asked. I knew right then and there that we were going to make a great team!

And Les had more surprises up his sleeve. He'd had his landscape architect redesign the building's courtyard to incorporate exercise and play equipment throughout. Under the new design, the courtyard resembled a hybrid circuit training course with art elements incorporated! Les also turned his community room into a gym with a children's climbing wall and exercise bikes with video games on their monitors to entice teens. And he transformed his rooftop into that hydroponic farm—the first of its kind on a residential building in the United States. Sky Vegetables would supply a percentage of the vegetables produced to building residents, and sell the rest to New York City restaurants and chefs who were keen on sourcing their food locally. The money from the sales would help to support the costs of the farm. Active Design affordable housing is one thing; Active Design affordable housing that also makes healthy food available in the middle of a food desert is something else altogether—something extraordinary.

But Les also presented us with another present at our second meeting. Although Les, Joyce, and I had discussed possible design improvements for Arbor House—actual construction was still several years out—Les told us that he had also asked his architect to do whatever was still possible to improve the completed designs of a project that would be built even sooner: The Melody. Les's insistence had led to his architect taking a hard look at what could be done and making new, last-minute modifications. In particular, building entrances could be changed to face the stairwells, bright paint could be added to drab and neglected spaces like the stairwells, and it wasn't too late to buy exercise equipment and play equipment for the community room and the backyards. In 2011, The Melody opened, accompanied by a *New York Times* story: "Bronx Apartment Building Designed to Combat Obesity."

Then, in 2013, Arbor House opened its doors, and the response was overwhelmingly positive. In addition to being platinum-certified by LEED, Arbor House was also recognized by the American Cancer Society as a "Healthy High-Rise," due to its completely smoke-free status. But perhaps the most important accolades came from the building's new residents. In a *TIME* magazine profile, Luis Giurias spoke about how the building's amenities were making a difference for him and for his family. He'd never exercised as a kid, he admitted, but he believes that Arbor House is setting his kids up for a lifetime of better health. "This will make it second nature to them to be healthy," he told *TIME*. "It won't be foreign to them like it was for me."

Addressing the Skeptics: The Affordable Housing Study

The Active Design movement was racking up success stories. The Riverside Health Center, Intervale Green, Via Verde, Arbor House, The Melody—all had affordably incorporated strategies (or were in the midst of doing so) from the Active Design Guidelines, and were using modifications that would qualify them for the LEED Innovation Credit for Physical Activity. Still, skeptics continued to cast doubt on the feasibility of routine integration of these strategies into affordable housing. "Via Verde is an exception," we would hear from affordable housing developers who hadn't given the strategies a chance. "It won a special competition. What about all the projects that don't win competitions? What about the costs involved for real-world building projects?"

As I continued to work with the New York City Department of Housing Preservation and Development (HPD), I heard again and again how the department could only wish that all developers were like Jonathan Rose and Blue Sea. So many other developers were utterly unconvinced that they could do what Via Verde, Arbor House and The Melody had done. Clearly, we needed to do something to convince them. I put forward an idea: What about a study to quantify the costs of integrating Active Design Guideline strategies into affordable housing? The HPD responded enthusiastically, agreeing both to partner with the health department and to bring on some additional affordable housing developers. Our study—*Active Design: Affordable Designs for Affordable Housing*—was off to the races.

Now Dr. Gayle Nicoll reminded me that the Robert Wood Johnson Foundation's Active Living Research (ALR) Program had put out a call for research proposals. Gayle and I agreed to apply jointly for one of the ALR grants. We brainstormed what study could best be done with the amount of funding available. We brainstormed what sites we could include, and what other partners we should invite. And we reached out to Dr. Craig Zimring, who was too busy to be involved directly but introduced us to his colleague Jennifer Dubose at the Georgia Institute of Technology, who agreed to jump in.

In the end, we proposed to undertake a study of affordable housing projects in each of our three cities: New York, San Antonio, Texas, and Atlanta, Georgia. Each of us would bring on board our city's affordable housing department or authority and a few affordable housing developers. Through a series of case studies, we would quantify the costs of building new affordable housing developments in each of the cities. Then, we would find recently built developments, determine their costs of construction, and redesign them according to Active Design Guideline strategies. We would re-cost them for the materials and equipment needed, and compare the new costs with the original development costs. We sent in our grant proposal just in the nick of time. It was a harrowing experience, hovering over our screens as the electronic upload system slowed to a snail's pace while it worked to receive all of the large files being sent by researchers across the country. We breathed a huge sigh of relief when the "Sent" confirmation finally popped up.

A few months later, Active Living Research responded—we were in! So began two years of hard work, two years of study that would confirm what we already knew from our ongoing work with the Riverside Health Center, Intervale Green, Via Verde, The Melody, and Arbor House: the integration of Active Design Guideline strategies into affordable housing developments had only a minimal effect on overall costs, to a maximum increased cost of 1.6 percent of the total development costs across eleven case study projects in the three cities. In fact, seven of the eleven case studies showed increased costs of only 0.01 to 0.6 percent—well under 1 percent—and one project even showed a cost *savings* by integrating the health-promoting strategies. Furthermore, with the help of the developer partners who had participated in the study with us, other feasibility concerns and considerations had also been addressed. At the end of the study, Gayle, Jennifer, and I were able to break down the available strategies into three categories: 1) low-cost, immediately implementable, and requiring minimal change to how affordable housing tends to already be designed; 2) no cost or minimal cost, but requiring modest changes to existing building designs, and; 3) more challenging, but still achievable if supported by market-rate tenant expectations (in mixed income developments, for example), operational budgets, and municipal policies.

The result of our work, the Affordable Housing study—which represented yet another accomplishment based on coordination across sectors—would become critical for the next phase of the Active Design movement. In this phase, Active Design Guidelines strategies supporting healthy choices for people in our buildings, streets, and neighborhoods would not be incorporated in an ad hoc manner but would become integrated routinely into the design and construction of these built environments. The Affordable Housing study would play a critical role in this initiative for buildings, particularly for affordable housing.

If You Build It . . .

Some might say that the story of the Active Design movement in New York has a happy ending—but I prefer to think of it as a happy beginning. On June 27, 2013, Mayor Michael Bloomberg signed an executive order for Active Design, supported by the Department of Citywide Administrative Services, the Department of Housing Preservation and Development, the Department of Design and Construction, and the Department of Transportation. Moving forward, City agencies would be required to review the design of all construction and major renovation projects to assess opportunities to implement Active Design elements in City buildings and streets. The order also required that agencies assess opportunities to promote the use of stairways, and train design and construction personnel in the use of the City's Active Design Guidelines.

Finally, we would have a systematic and routine integration of strategies to promote physical activity in all City design and construction projects, just as the integration of sanitation and clean water into all our buildings was made systematic in centuries past to prevent and control infectious diseases. This was what I had been asked to do when I came to New York in 2006: to bring about change that would encode modifications to our human-made environments that support the prevention of chronic diseases like heart disease, stroke, common and deadly cancers like colon cancer, and diabetes, and their major risk factors of obesity and physical inactivity.

It had taken nearly eight years, and more work than I could ever have imagined, but the results, too, had exceeded my expectations. What had started as a brainstorming session back at that first Fit City conference had become a movement, and that movement had inspired action, both in New York and farther afield. I had had the pleasure of seeing Active Design come to life in projects like the Riverside Health Center, Intervale Green, The Melody, Arbor House, and Via Verde. I had seen New Yorkers embrace opportunities to take stairs instead of elevators, and to squeeze in a workout or a walk on their lunch hour, or before or after work. I'd heard from many of them about their frustrations with a lack of access to facilities that encouraged a more active lifestyle. And I'd met so many like-minded people—men and women who had come to Fit City conferences to learn and discuss, or who sought out the Active Design Guidelines to see what they might be able to do in their own cities. It hadn't been easy, but we'd made progress. And along the way, I had met some incredibly talented and dedicated people, and even had some fun! No doubt, there was still work to be done—there were so many buildings in the city beyond what was owned, constructed and operated by the City of New York, for starters—but I felt optimistic about my "happy beginning," and the places it might lead in the years to come. And on that day in June, as I read the press coverage of Mayor Bloomberg's executive order, I couldn't help but recall the movie *Field of Dreams*, and its now famous line: "If you build it, they will come." Indeed.

PART THREE

HOW WE MOVE

It's no secret that active living is a key part of our overall health. Whether we're talking about weight loss or mobility or cardiovascular fitness or even prevention of cancers like colon cancer, the message is clear: the more we move, the better off we are.

Given this basic truth, it's painful for me to see cities, suburbs, and developments growing seemingly without awareness of the problems they will inevitably encounter as a result of their inattention to how we move. By now, one of these problems should be sounding awfully familiar: an increasingly unhealthy population, with ever-rising rates of noncontagious diseases such as diabetes and cancers, and their risk factors of obesity and physical inactivity.

But it doesn't stop there. When the places we live in are constructed without a conscious intention to offer more opportunities for physical activity—whether that comes in service of getting from Point A to Point B, or as part of the recreation that is so important to our emotional and physical health—we are setting ourselves up for a host of related problems. What happens to our older citizens when they can no longer drive themselves to stores or doctor's appointments or the homes of relatives and friends? What happens to businesses when that same population can no longer easily pop in for a quick shop? What happens to our cities when traffic congestion is so bad that it prevents people from wanting to live or do business there? And what happens to the environment when our overwhelming reliance on the automobile continues to wreak havoc?

And yet, day after day after day, governments and organizations around the world continue to make urban-planning choices that prioritize cars over people, so that residents who want to choose a healthier lifestyle must overcome daunting obstacles or make superhuman commitments. Public funds are poured into the construction of new highways, and not into subway extensions or other rapid transit options. Parking lots are constructed where playgrounds or green spaces might have been created. Bike lanes are rejected in favor of road land expansions. And suburbs continue to be designed with acre after acre of single-family homes, situated beyond walking distance from the nearest amenities and with no other options for people to move to as they age.

But it's not too late to change. Although the negative effects of climate change are now already being felt on a daily basis (in the form of extreme weather events such as heat waves, floods, tornadoes, and freak winter storms), the hope is that if we act now we will at least be able to mitigate the severity of these events going forward. The same is true for our health outcomes. We need to act now. We need to do what we can to ensure that people can make the lifestyle choices that will help them to stay healthy—and independent—longer. We need to help people get and stay active, goals they themselves are setting yearly at New Year's and then usually failing miserably.

There are hopeful signs. We've seen a growing recognition of the importance of play in our daily lives, regardless of age. And we've seen the birth of movements dedicated to replacing our old, unhealthy patterns with better ones. Smart Growth, New Urbanism, Transit-Oriented Development, Active Design—all are focused on finding different, healthier ways to develop and grow our cities, ways that will enable us to embrace a more active and healthy lifestyle, and maintain it over time. This kind of work is not easy, but it's not impossible. As is so often the case, it takes a combination of vision, creativity, determination, and cooperation.

7 | PRIORITIZING PEOPLE

CREATING CHOICES FOR ACTIVE TRANSPORTATION

MY FATHER AND I are walking. We're heading to the bank across the street from the condo where my parents live. You have to be over fifty-five years old to be the primary residents in their building, and many of them are seniors like my parents. After the bank, my father and I need to cross the street again to the supermarket for groceries and the pharmacy to pick up birthday cards for my mother.

My parents live on the northwest side of Edmonton, Alberta, not far by car to the famous West Edmonton Mall, once the world's largest shopping mall and still number one in North America. Edmonton is a city that used to be cold and snowy, without fail, from the end of October through at least March or April, before climate change turned those patterns into less predictable ones. My mother's birthday is at the end of November, and I am in Edmonton to celebrate it with her. I'm looking forward to her birthday dinner, which is bound to include Peking duck, a family favorite for special occasions. I'm already dreaming of crispy cara-melized duck skin served with warm, thin crepes and shredded scallions, duck bone soup with vegetables, and deboned duck meat stir-fried with Chinese greens.

As my father and I wait for a break in traffic to cross the street, I find myself thinking that my parents are, in a way, very lucky. They can walk to the bank, the supermarket, and the pharmacy, if absolutely necessary. But I know they rarely make these trips on foot—it's just a five-minute walk to the bank, but it means crossing a four-lane road packed with quickly moving cars, as my father and I are doing now. He had offered to drive me, and when I'd opted instead for some fresh air and walking he'd reluctantly agreed to tag along. There's a traffic light some distance away, at the next intersection, but as we crunch along the snowy sidewalk my father tells me that a pedestrian was killed at that very intersection not long ago.

Banking done, we cross the same street at the intersection with the traffic light. At eighty-three, my father is still spry, but he is concerned that a day will soon come when he won't be able to walk fast enough to cross that four-lane road, especially with the traffic light timed for a young-adult pace. He worries, too, that failing eyesight might prevent him from driving, and then how would he and my mother get around? How would they buy groceries and birthday cards? How would they go to the bank? "How would we go see your brother, and our grandchildren, and our friends?" he asks. Would they have to move to a long-term care facility or nursing home, even if they could otherwise care for themselves?

My father and mother are not alone in this concern. These are the dilemmas faced by those who are aging in many of our cities and communities around the world. Car-focused, car-dominated, car-only cities and neighborhoods are excluding many of our citizens—not just seniors but also children, teens, parents with strollers, and those who cannot or choose not to own a car—from being able to fully and easily participate in healthy, independent living. These same cities and neighborhoods are also making many of us overweight or obese, and contributing to our ongoing weight gain.

Decades ago, before cars became our primary mode of transportation, we were much more active. We walked or cycled to
places. Many of our jobs involved some sort of activity—not
just parking ourselves in front of a computer from nine to five,
or beyond. Our kids played outside, not in front of screens. And
we were healthier for it, with much lower rates of the noncontagious diseases that are now running rampant. These days, it's a
different story. Physical inactivity contributes to 3.2 million deaths
annually around the world—3.2 million *preventable* deaths. That's
about a tenth of the entire population of Canada, every year.
Studies conducted in the United States have shown that, despite
the adult population self-reporting that they get an average of
392 minutes of physical activity a week, when people wore physical activity devices called accelerometers, their weekly moderate-
to vigorous-intensity activity was shown to be only 47 minutes per
week. That true figure is well below the recommendations of the
U.S. Department of Health and Human Services to get at least
75 minutes of vigorous-intensity, or 150 minutes of moderate-
intensity physical activity per week to maintain and improve health.

A recent and extensive New York City measurement study,
using both accelerometers and GPS tracking devices, found that
adults there averaged 118 minutes of at least moderate-intensity
physical activity weekly, getting two and a half times more measured physical activity than the rest of the country (although
New Yorkers still fell short of the 150-minute recommendations).
When measured by the accelerometers, 23 percent of New
Yorkers were completely inactive (defined as not having a single
ten-minute bout of moderate to vigorous-intensity physical activity during the week), compared to the majority of Americans.

What's going on in New York? How are those New Yorkers
getting so many more minutes of physical activity than the rest of
the country? One of the study's key findings is that these men
and women didn't tend to go to the gym, and they didn't rely on

having a regular exercise routine. Only 17.5 percent of the reported minutes of physical activity among New Yorkers were coming from recreational exercise. Instead, they got their physical activity mostly by walking around town, doing what they needed to get done in everyday life—getting to work, running errands, attending social events, and so on. That's proof positive that it doesn't take a lot to make a difference, and that solutions to this modern-day dilemma of ill health and inactivity could be closer at hand than we think.

Walk This Way: Taking Steps Toward a Healthier Future

Physical activity and public health experts today emphasize active living rather than intentional exercise to help people achieve the physical activity needed for health in daily life. Everyday daily transportation needs can often provide the best opportunity for people to incorporate the ten-minute bouts of physical activity that are optimal for health, without the extra time commitment required to go to the gym or for a run, plans that usually fail to compete against the regular demands of life. If you are able to walk your children to school and then walk yourself to work (and repeat that routine in reverse at the end of the day), and walk to get healthy food or just to stretch your legs at lunch, these minutes can add up, helping you to achieve that 150 minutes or more of moderate-intensity physical activity a week. If you accumulated a mere thirty minutes a day every weekday, you wouldn't have to worry that you missed the gym again. A ten-minute walk to school, then to work, and then to lunch, and back again, would help you achieve sixty minutes of walking each weekday—double the physical activity recommendations for adults. For children, this type of daily walking is an important complement to physical education and active play, since their activity needs for health are even higher: 60 minutes of moderate- to vigorous-intensity physical activity every day, amounting to 420 minutes a week.

When it comes to promoting the notion that more transportation should be *active* transportation—that is, walking and cycling—studies now show that street and neighborhood features make a huge difference. Where the choice to walk, cycle, or take public transit (which often starts and ends with a walk) is readily available, safe, convenient, and pleasant, people are making that choice. Even the design of buildings and how they interface with our streets can matter.

A number of key publications have synthesized the issues related to walkability. After an evidence review completed in 2004, now a decade and a half ago, the U.S. Department of Health and Human Services' Guide to Community Preventive Services published a new recommendation for increasing physical activity, updated from its 2001 findings. Led by Dr. Greg Heath, the 2004 review concluded that there was sufficient scientific evidence for recommending community- and street-scale urban design and land-use policies as important interventions for increasing physical activity. At the street level, the authors concluded, policies involving building codes, road design standards, and environmental changes are important. Street design features that are associated with increased physical activity include safety elements such as improved street lighting; projects that work toward safe pedestrian crossings; features that calm traffic, like street humps and traffic circles; and features that improve the aesthetic environment for walking, such as improved landscaping. These features, the reviewers found, could increase physical activity by a median of 35 percent.

Community design features and policies are also important. Locating residential zones close to stores, schools, jobs, and recreation areas facilitates walking, as long as there is also a safe and pleasant way to do so. For example, effective design connects people from their homes to nearby amenities on good sidewalks using the shortest routes possible on grid-pattern streets (rather than the lollipop loops leading nowhere that are so common in suburban cul-de-sacs), good lighting, safe street crossings, and nice landscaping are design elements that signal to a walker that the experience will be both safe and pleasant. Greg Heath and his co-authors found that policies—including those governing zoning codes, building codes, and building practices—could be used to create better environmental conditions. Community-scale designs and policies that improved neighborhood features, the authors found, could improve physical activity by a median of 161 percent.

Before beginning his current work as Guerry Professor of Exercise Science at the University of Tennessee, Chattanooga campus, Greg Heath was leader of the Interventions Team in the CDC's Physical Activity and Health Branch. Like so many of his colleagues, Greg wanted the growing research on physical activity to be translated into actionable policies and practices. During my time there as a disease detective, I found myself in his office frequently for discussions, both prior to and after the environmental assessments conducted in West Virginia.

The West Virginia assessments confirmed much of what was being discussed about the potential impact of physical activity interventions—or the consequences when those interventions aren't present. Remember that a third of the road segments around the schools we audited in Clarksburg-Bridgeport had no sidewalks, while the streets around worksites were even worse, with 90 percent lacking sidewalks. In rural Gilmer County, less than 10 percent of the road segments around schools had sidewalks, and not a single street segment around the largest worksites in the county had a sidewalk, even though housing was located nearby and 40 percent of the road segments were deemed to be busy streets. And at the time of our investigation, West Virginia was ranked third among U.S. states for obesity, second for diabetes and first for high blood pressure. It's not a stretch here to connect the dots.

Unfortunately, these conditions aren't unique to the small cities and rural counties of West Virginia. They exist all across North America, and around the world. No wonder, then, that most of us find it a challenge to get in that daily activity we so badly need. No wonder that our health markers are worsening with every passing year.

I had the good fortune to arrive at my post in New York City's Department of Health and Mental Hygiene as the world was waking up to the connection between the built environment and our health—a time when some forward-thinking governments were beginning to see that they had a role to play in stopping the spread of obesity and its related conditions. Several movements devoted to greener—and healthier—urban development and design were on the rise. The Smart Growth development theory was encouraging a mix of building types and uses; diverse housing and transportation options; development within existing, high-density neighborhoods; and community engagement. The higher population density that usually comes with mixing in a range of housing options (as opposed to an overabundance of single-family homes) is often a prerequisite for having enough people to support nearby businesses. In turn, those businesses—connected to each other and to residential areas with sidewalks and bicycle lanes—serve as motivation, and support, for safe, active, non-automobile transportation. For its part, the New Urbanism design philosophy promotes walkable communities by including a variety of housing types and a variety of non-residential amenities nearby. And Transit-Oriented Development adds public transit integration into Smart Growth planning and New Urbanist designs.

The proponents of these movements and others—such as the Active Design movement—are well aware of our poor health markers, and the reasons behind them; as they take on roles in various levels of government and non-governmental organizations, more and more cities and counties are committing to change. In places both large and small, urban and rural, strategies are now being employed to improve support for more active modes of transportation—be it walking, biking, or public transit—with some unexpected and encouraging results.

Big Changes in the Big Apple

Janette Sadik-Khan is tall, slim, outspoken, and formidable. Appointed by Mayor Michael Bloomberg as New York City's Transportation commissioner in 2007, Janette immediately went to work instituting the changes that were needed to create choices that would support all road users: pedestrians, cyclists, transit users, and drivers. Asked by the mayor during her interview why she wanted to be "traffic commissioner" for the City of New York, Janette answered that she didn't, in fact, want to be a traffic commissioner. "I want to be a *transportation* commissioner," she said. When her answer was met with silence, Janette figured she'd blown it. She was wrong. As it turned out, Mayor Bloomberg's silence was thoughtful. She was hired soon after.

The same year that Janette was hired, New York City released PlaNYC 2030—the master plan that identified goals for an environmentally sustainable and livable city in 2030, anticipating a population growth of roughly a million new residents. A key goal was to ensure the availability of enough modes of transportation to prevent the introduction of a million more cars onto New York City's already congested streets.

The municipal government's commitment to PlaNYC 2030 helped Janette, during her tenure at the Department of Transportation (DOT), to lead nothing short of a transformation of the city's streets: the addition of nearly four hundred miles of bike lanes, along with a dramatic increase in the number of racks; the creation of the first parking-protected bike lanes in North America (with bike paths situated between the sidewalk and the protection of a parked car, rather than between parked and moving cars, as is so often the case); and the redesign of hundreds of intersections and streets in a successful effort to decrease traffic fatalities. And that's just scratching the surface.

Seeking out successful transportation and public space ideas from around the world, Janette brought them to New York City and championed their implementation through tireless work across departments, proving yet again that cooperation is the key to progress when it comes to public health and public policy interventions. In 2008, the launch of the city's first Bus Rapid Transit (BRT) lines—the Select Bus Service—was the culmination of work between the DOT and the Metropolitan Transportation Authority.

New York City is well known for its subway system. A large number of interconnected lines can take you to many places within the five boroughs that make up the city. Because of this, it was often assumed that public transportation options were adequate. In fact, nothing could have been further from the truth. Rather than offering transportation to everyone, a reliance on subway and local bus meant that there were many people who were inadequately served by rapid public transit. Local buses are often stuck in congested traffic; they make stops at every light or intersection to let people on and off. This is highly frustrating for the many people who rely on them, notably young people, like students, and workers who can't afford to live at or near a subway stop. And though expanding the subway system is always a possibility, the reality is that such expansions of rail systems can be both prolonged and extremely expensive. A faster, less expensive option was needed. Janette turned to examples from countries who couldn't afford the more expensive rail options, countries like Colombia and Brazil. Cities like Bogotá had for several decades relied on Bus Rapid Transit as a cheap, fast transit option.

The Select Bus Service in New York City was designed to improve the public transit experience on two fronts: by reducing travel time, and by increasing the comfort level for customers. The system supplements existing bus service in areas under-served by the subway, such as the far east side of Manhattan (First and Second Avenues), some busy streets in the Bronx, and many parts of Staten Island. New buses, routes, and stops were created, along with clearly marked bus-only lanes—complete with cameras to catch drivers who might consider using one to sneak past a traffic jam. The stops are farther apart, catering to users who need to go farther faster than the local bus service would allow. Each stop features ticket-purchasing machines, eliminating the need to pay the driver when you board, and the buses are equipped with all-door boarding to further decrease the time spent at stops. The Traffic Signal Priority system was also implemented, giving the buses priority at traffic lights.

The Select Bus Service was clearly a step forward in terms of decreasing traffic congestion and encouraging public transit use, but what about physical activity? How much physical activity, in the form of walking, were Select Bus Service users getting compared to local bus users? Seeking to answer that question, I enlisted the help of Dr. Kristen Day and her class of undergraduate students at New York University's Polytechnic University. Kristen was an urban planning professor there, and she agreed to collaborate with me on this study. With a questionnaire that Kristen and I had co-created in hand, the students would wait at designated Select Bus Service stops, and at designated local bus stops on the same streets. The students would "intercept" waiting passengers and, if they agreed to participate, ask them questions related to their walking to the bus stop. What we learned was that, thanks to the much greater distance between stops for the Select Bus Service compared to the local bus stops, Select Bus Service riders had more walking compared to local bus riders. Although there was variation across study participants, those using the Select Bus Service appeared to get, on average, an extra half a block of walking compared with local bus riders. Although this may not seem like much, large east-west city blocks in New York City can take four minutes to walk across. Thus, accumulating an extra half block of walking regularly, every single day, perhaps multiple times a day for regular users, could really contribute toward the 150 minutes of weekly physical activity that people need to get. By providing more transit options *and* better health outcomes, the Select Bus Service was a win-win. But it was just one of many DOT initiatives to help get more New Yorkers moving.

Wendy Feuer is taking questions. It's October 2012, and she and I are in Mississauga, Ontario, for the Healthy Peel by Design conference, which has brought together health and non-health professionals from the region's three municipalities. We've talked about environmental supports for healthy living, and shared some of the successes we've achieved in New York, including many that improve the ability of residents to build activity into their day-to-day lives. As it turns out, the audience is particularly curious about just that.

One attendee raises her hand: "Has the New York City Department of Transportation ever encountered public opposition to the bike lanes and pedestrian plazas constructed during Mayor Michael Bloomberg's administration?"

As one of Janette Sadik-Khan's assistant commissioners at the New York City Department of Transportation, Wendy is more than qualified to answer that question. I listen as she admits that it's not always easy to put in bike lanes or new pedestrian plazas, even in New York. "But it's worth it," she continues. "We really have to do it. Why? Because a safe city is a healthy city is a competitive city."

Eager to back up her assertion with facts, Wendy flips through her slides to one she'd presented earlier: a picture of Times

Square in midtown Manhattan. Famous for decades for its theater district and Broadway shows, Times Square has become famous in recent years for another reason: the creation of a pedestrian plaza in one of the most traffic-congested areas in New York. In 2009 the Department of Transportation, with support from Mayor Bloomberg and the Department of Health and Mental Hygiene, began an experiment. Certain streets in Times Square would be closed to cars and opened up for use only by pedestrians. If the results being gathered on traffic flow, retail sales, air pollution, injuries, and pedestrian counts moved in a negative direction, the experiment could quickly be stopped.

Despite some healthy skepticism, the experiment was a resounding success. Instead of a downturn, as some retailers had feared, sales shot through the roof and propelled Times Square onto a list of the world's top ten retail areas. Traffic flow was managed well by reprogramming traffic-light signals and diverting cars appropriately to surrounding streets. Air pollution levels dropped. Pedestrian counts increased. Injuries to pedestrians dropped *and* injuries to motorists dropped even more.

The City needed to know what impacts its innovations—the pedestrian plaza, bicycle lanes, Select Bus Service—were having. In 2012, the DOT compiled this data, and the data collected at multiple intervention sites across the five boroughs of New York City, in *Measuring the Street: New Metrics for 21st Century Streets*. Drawing on recent successes, the report described key approaches to street-design projects and showed how the results could improve city streets for all users, from pedestrians to cyclists to public transit users to drivers. On Eighth and Ninth Avenues on the west side of Manhattan, where the first protected bicycle lanes in the United States were implemented, data showed a 35 to 58 percent decrease in injuries to all users, along with a 49 percent increase in retail sales. Traffic-calming measures on East 180th Street in the Bronx led to decreases in speeding and a 67 percent reduction in pedestrian crashes. Around Union Square, expansion of the pedestrian spaces and inclusion of protected bicycle lanes was followed by decreased speeding, fewer pedestrian collisions, and a 49 percent drop in commercial space vacancies. Converting an underused parking area into a pedestrian plaza on Pearl Street in Brooklyn increased retail sales in the area by 172 percent. Improving bus routes on Fordham Road in the Bronx resulted in a 10 percent increase in bus ridership, a 20 percent improvement in bus speeds, and a 71 percent increase in retail sales. Improving pedestrian spaces, bicycle lanes, and traffic signals and timings on Hoyt Avenue in Queens resulted in an improvement in travel times, a decrease in travel collisions, and an increase in bicycle volumes. And so, from the data, we knew that people were using many transportation modes to get to these locations. From retail sales and such going up, we knew people were embracing the idea of walking to do errands, to shop, to enjoy the city. And that meant more activity, with an attendant improvement in people's health and in the health of our businesses.

Thanks in large part to efforts championed by the Department of Transportation under the leadership of Janette Sadik-Kahn—and supported by many other departments, organizations, and community groups—New York was fast becoming a much more pedestrian-friendly city. But in 2013, it took yet another step in the right direction—or perhaps "pedal" would be a better word.

In May 2013, New York City launched Citi Bike, the largest bike-share program in the country. Inspired by great cycling cities in Europe, like Amsterdam and Copenhagen, Janette had already overseen the DOT's installation of numerous bicycle racks and the implementation of protected bike lanes. On the west side of Manhattan, perched between the West Side Highway and the scenic Hudson River, a new shared-use greenway now stretched the length of the island, offering people a space to bicycle on an off-road path, or to rollerblade, run, or walk. By teaming up with the Department of Parks and Recreation, the greenway is now also flanked in many parts by new city parks, basketball courts, tennis courts, and even kayaking stations constructed on old abandoned piers and areas under highways and alongside old railway tracks, that provide recreation opportunities for those with the time to stop on their cycling, walking, or rollerblading route.

The bike-share program was a logical extension of the city's infrastructure improvements for safer bicycling. If London, Paris, Dublin, Montreal, and Washington, D.C., could have a bike-share program, why not New York? Citi Bike features a fleet of specially designed, sturdy bikes that are locked into docking stations located throughout the city. Riders can pick up a bike from one station and return it to any other station, making them an ideal option for one-way trips. They can be used to commute, to run errands, or to enjoy a bit of weekend or evening recreation.

New Yorkers seemed more than ready to embrace the idea. Weeks before the program launched, five thousand founding memberships had sold out. Since then, the program has steadily expanded, adding additional bikes and docking stations. In October 2017, Citi Bike riders logged their fifty-millionth trip—proving yet again that when supports for healthy living exist and are safe and well-designed, people are generally eager to use them.

Buses and Bikes in Bogotá

The work done by the Department of Transportation during the Bloomberg administration was inspired, in some ways, by initiatives playing out far from New York's bustling streets. One of Janette Sadik-Kahn's skills was her ability to look beyond borders for great transportation and public space ideas. She would come across ingenious ideas and then work with her staff and others to incorporate them into New York City.

Like New York, Bogotá, Colombia, is a major metropolitan hub. Home to upwards of eight million people, it too has been a leader in thinking outside the box when it comes to supports for both public transportation and increased physical activity (see chapter 8 to learn more about the city's *ciclovía* and *recreovía*). In this busy urban center, many residents are poor; some cannot afford to own a car, and for many who can, the associated costs are a challenge.

Bogotá has found three major ways to deal with these issues, some more successful than others. First, the city developed the TransMilenio rapid transit system. Red buses run along dedicated lanes in the middle of city streets, between well-spaced stations. Unimpeded by the congested car traffic in the other lanes, these buses move quickly, offering residents an affordable, speedy option for getting where they need to go. The TransMilenio has been wildly successful. Other North American cities, like Mexico City, have adopted similar systems. And more affluent cities with traffic congestion and air pollution issues like New York and Los Angeles are also looking to Bogotá to learn. In Canada, Toronto and Quebec City have started to create their own Bus Rapid Transit routes. Expansion talks in Bogotá are also in the works, with hopes of addressing the issue of increasingly crowded buses.

While affordable and fast public transit was a key tool in Bogotá's approach to its transportation issues, members of the city government knew that they also had to deal with cars. If you ever find yourself on a Bogotá street, check out the license plates on the cars around you. They don't all look the same; in fact, there appear to be two different color schemes. And no, it's not because the city is letting drivers coordinate colors with their favorite soccer team. The color coding is one way that the city is managing its traffic congestion. One color means you're allowed to drive in the city on Mondays, Wednesdays, and Fridays. With the other color, you're allowed on the road on Tuesdays and

Thursdays. The result? Only half the number of cars on the road on any given weekday. Unfortunately, the roads are still congested. And because no such rules exist on the weekend, weekend driving too is highly congested in Bogotá. The alternating license plates designating allowed days of driving has also been implemented in other traffic-congested cities from which Bogotá may have gotten the idea, such as Mexico City.

Bogotá continues to look for solutions that could concurrently improve traffic congestion and provide opportunities for physical activity. The city has started to expand its network of off-road bicycle lanes to serve as safe, viable options for transportation. Though these bicycle lanes are safe from car traffic, the people in Bogotá I've spoken with tell me they are not necessarily safe from crime. During the World Health Organization's Pan American Health Organization conference in 2012, one city government member told me: "I know many people who are afraid that they might get robbed on a bicycle on these off-road bicycle lanes, especially since these bike paths are not so busy right now." It's the vicious but unavoidable interconnection of safety and numbers. To attract more users, the bike paths need to feel safe. But to feel safe, the bike paths need to attract more users. In a consultation session, I suggested that programming and activities could perhaps be used to attract more users, and that perhaps the lanes needed to be protected from car traffic but located on the roads, where there are more watchful eyes to create a feeling of safety.

Multiple Choice

Of course, the availability of bike lanes, good public transportation, and safe sidewalks does more than get us moving; it also gives people choices. We've seen the studies showing that U.S. households in completely automobile-dependent neighborhoods spend on average 25 percent of their monthly income on transportation-related costs, while in neighborhoods with a variety of transportation choices, including mass transit, that number drops to 9 percent, freeing up money to address other, critical needs. But the issues around transportation choice go beyond money. For many seniors, including my parents, what's at stake in having transportation choices beyond the automobile is independent living. Can they walk or bus to where they'll need to go in order to get their physical and social needs met once they stop driving?

Given the intermingled concerns over health, affordability, and independence, it's not surprising that surveys are increasingly showing that people want to live in communities and neighborhoods where a variety of transportation modes and amenities are available within walking distance. In the United States, polls conducted by the National Association of Realtors show that Smart Growth communities are gaining in popularity, compared to communities defined by urban sprawl. In fact, the majority of those polled since 2011 said they wanted to live in communities that feature a mix of housing types; where streets have sidewalks; where there are restaurants, shopping, libraries, and schools close enough to walk to as well as drive to; and where there is public transportation nearby. Similar studies have been undertaken by the Australian Heart Foundation and have shown even more people—the vast majority—preferring to live in neighborhoods that support a variety of amenities and transportation choices. Even in Edmonton—the most sprawled city in Canada—surveys conducted by the municipal government revealed a desire for walkable access to public transportation, and to amenities such as schools, libraries, restaurants, shopping, and recreation opportunities.

Perhaps people are intuitively coming around to the same conclusions that public health officials, urban planners, and urban designers have already drawn in recent years: life is better when we don't have to rely only on cars to get us everywhere we need to go. Stretching our legs a few times a day feels good, and is clearly good for us, for our cities, for the environment, and even for our businesses. Given those outcomes—and provided the right supports are in place—it's hard not to be inspired to walk to work, to bike to the bank, or to tack a quick stroll onto the end of your evening public transit commute. Before you know it, you'll have racked up that 150 minutes of weekly physical activity you need to maintain and improve your health.

8 | EMBRACING PLAY

MOVING FOR THE FUN OF IT

IT IS 8:20 A.M. on a weekday and I'm at a public school in a wealthy suburb of New Jersey. Not a single child here has walked to school, not even the ones who live next door. In much of the town, there are no sidewalks.

Every morning, the school's occupational therapist runs a special class for the kindergarteners in the lunchroom, which also functions as the school's all-purpose room. The gray laminate tables where the children will eat have been folded up and placed along the walls. Fluorescent lighting shines from the ceiling, mixing with the sunlight coming in through two large windows on the back wall. Long gray curtains hang on each side of the windows.

The children's homeroom teacher enters the room. Her charges file in behind her, one by one. Johnny walks straight as an arrow, with Radhika following. Alexei is behind her, out of line and looking at the ceiling. Next comes Joan. She barely lifts her feet as she takes her small steps, appearing lethargic despite the fact that she's only five years old and it's first thing in the morning. And on and on, until eighteen students have entered and taken a seat on the floor facing the therapist and teacher.

The class begins. The occupational therapist tells the children they are going to learn how to crawl like a baby and walk like a bear. She asks for a volunteer to do the bear walk. Radhika's arm shoots straight up. She puts her hands to the floor, straightens her legs behind her, and moves herself forward without letting her knees touch the ground. The next two children who try are not as successful. They are uncoordinated. They don't have enough strength. In fact, about half the children are unable to do the bear walk.

It is for exactly these reasons that the school introduced this class a few years ago. We live in an age when many children spend much of their time playing inactively on screens and tablets. Children who play predominantly on such devices are losing touch with the spontaneous jumping, running, crawling, tree-climbing, throwing, and digging that came with active play and being outside And they might need to be taught again how to play actively with their bodies, using gross motor skills. They may also need help developing their fine motor skills. Since some of the children are no longer outside playing in the sandbox, no longer picking up pieces of toys or insects or sticks and stones with their fingers and thumbs, they have trouble picking up their pencils and erasers. The next morning, the occupational therapist has them practice picking up small balls and blocks that they then place in a cup.

This is the state of children's play today. The transition from active outdoor and indoor play to increasingly sedentary, screen-based activities is negatively affecting our children's health. Not so long ago, we equated screen time with television viewing; these days, it also includes time spent on computers, tablets, smartphones, and other electronic devices. Today, more than 30 percent of children in the United States and Canada are overweight or obese. As Bill Dietz's research has shown since 1985, and as other research has confirmed, television viewing and screen time are associated with obesity in children. According to statistics provided by the ParticipACTION program in Canada, today, 95 percent of children do not meet the daily physical activity recommendation for sixty minutes of moderate- to vigorous-intensity activity. And their parents are not exactly setting a good example. Adults, too, spend more time on screens than outside, more time sitting than walking. According to ParticipACTION, an estimated 85 percent of Canadian adults do not meet the adult physical activity recommendation of 150 moderate-intensity activity (or 75 vigorous-intensity) minutes per week.

The bottom line is this: we all need to move more. And one of the easiest ways we can do that is by embracing play—by getting out into the world on bikes, on rollerblades, or just on our own two feet; by fitting recreational activity into our day-to-day lives; and by taking that very necessary time to have a bit of fun. Unfortunately, this isn't always easy to do. Many cities don't have safe or accessible recreation areas. Parks and playgrounds are too few and too far between. Bike paths are poorly maintained, or precariously positioned along the sides of busy streets designed only for fast-moving cars. Green spaces are hard to come by in cities already full to bursting with buildings. For city planners and designers, public health professionals and community groups, it's a challenge, to be sure. We want our cities to support a good quality of life, to encourage healthy lifestyles, but how do we make that happen when space is at such a premium?

Well, as I've seen so often since I began this work, where there's a will, there's almost always a way.

Taking It to the Streets

I'm excited about this trip to Bogotá, though a bit nervous about my wardrobe selection. As soon as the plane touches down, I notice that the residents of this Latin American city—perched nearly nine thousand feet above sea level—are wearing leather or even down-filled jackets. Unlike the tropical beach cities not so far away, Bogotá's air is dry and cool. I wonder if I've brought a warm enough coat.

It's October 2012, and I'm in town to deliver a keynote address at a conference organized by the Pan American Health Organization (PAHO) for delegates from several Latin American countries. Because of our success in implementing innovative policies and programs for improving the built environment and chronic non-communicable diseases in New York City—and the resultant reversals in childhood obesity and increases in life expectancy, among other favorable outcomes for businesses, safety, and pollution—my New York colleagues and I have been getting more and more invitations from organizations around the world that want to hear about this work. Given that my Spanish is less than fluent, I am grateful for the two-way translation services PAHO is providing: we won't necessarily be speaking the same language, but we'll all understand each other.

I'm always happy to speak to other public health professionals about the work that we do. But there's something else I'm eager to check out in the Colombian capital—the famous *ciclovía* and *recreovía* that I've heard so much about over the years. Okay, "famous" might be an overstatement as far as the general population is concerned, but it's completely accurate for those of us working in the realm of physical activity and non-communicable diseases, and among the increasing number of cities around the world that are adopting the concept for their own streets.

Bogotá's *ciclovía*—or "bike way"—dates back to the 1970s, when a group of local cycling enthusiasts successfully lobbied to have certain main streets closed to traffic, and open to bikes, on set days and times. The idea got a boost in 1976 when Mayor Luis Prieto Ocampo made the *ciclovía* an official municipal program, promoted by the city's transportation department, and again in 1998 with the election of Enrique Peñalosa, a young, energetic mayor who supported the idea that citizens, not cars, should own the city's streets, at least for one day each week. Peñalosa once stated that "a citizen on a $30 bicycle is equally important to one in a $30,000 car"—music to the ears of public health professionals everywhere! On taking office in 1998, Peñalosa cancelled plans for a new highway and invested the money instead in bike lanes and the city's TransMilenio rapid transit system.

These days, the *ciclovía* is alive and well. Every Sunday, and on public holidays as well, Bogotá closes approximately seventy miles of roads to motor vehicles from 7:00 a.m. to 2:00 p.m. During these times, about a million of the city's eight million residents can be found out and about on the *ciclovía*, in one way or another. Some cycle, of course. Others walk or rollerblade. Some are on their way to one of the thirty or so free *recreovía*, or recreation stations, set up along the route by Bogotá's recreation department.

On this particular Sunday, my group gathers at the edge of a large public park where a *recreovía* has been set up. There's an instructor on stage with a boombox, and the music is blaring. For a while, I watch as a large group takes part in an aerobics class, smiles on their flushed faces. I turn to check out the street behind me. It's packed with cyclists, runners, rollerbladers, and parents pushing strollers. Some have the determined look of an athlete in training. Others are strolling and rolling along at a leisurely pace, enjoying conversations. Car traffic is relegated to the other side of the median, where what would normally be two lanes of one-way traffic has been converted to one lane each of two-way traffic. Military trainees and volunteers assist with the street closures, making sure things run smoothly. Never one to let an opportunity pass, I suggest to my guide—who works with the city's health department—that more attention might be paid to the many stands along the route, which sell beverages so high in calories and sugar that they largely negate the calories being burned by the physical activities.

Bogotá may have been one of the first places in the world to embrace the possibility of something like the *ciclovía*—a low-cost innovation that allows people to move more and in better ways—but the idea has spread. These days, similar initiatives can be found in, among other places, Australia, Argentina, Brazil, Belgium, Canada, India, Mexico, and the United States.

For the past decade, New York City has run a *ciclovía*-like event of its own. Inspired by what she saw in Bogotá and elsewhere, Transportation commissioner Janette Sadik-Kahn worked with numerous government departments and partners—including City Planning, Building, Sanitation, Health, and the NYC Fire and Police Departments, to name a few—and got the buy-in and cooperation she needed to launch Summer Streets.

On three consecutive Saturdays in August 2008, approximately seven miles of Park Avenue were closed to cars, allowing walkers, runners, cyclists, and families to experience this main thoroughfare in an entirely new way. From the Brooklyn Bridge to Seventy-Second Street on the Upper East Side, people cycled and rollerbladed, scootered and skateboarded, or just walked along, taking it all in and stopping at the recreation stations set up along the way. Kids played on climbing walls or splashed in dumpster pools. In tunnels under Grand Central Station usually reserved for cars, art installations drew excited crowds. Free bike rentals, free exercise classes, and jump-rope competitions took place along the route, while mini tennis courts were set up for children by laying down artificial turf over the pavement. It was truly an event that celebrated active transportation and play, and it was a roaring success. That first year, fifty thousand people took part in Summer Streets. In 2016, that figure was closer to three hundred thousand.

In the busy days before the event launched, however, we had no idea what to expect. The Department of Transportation knew from the very early stages of planning that it wanted to assess attendance, traffic flows, and economic impacts. I was curious about that too, but I had my own list of questions. Topping that list: What kind of impact could Summer Streets have on health, particularly physical activity? I asked the DOT if we could work together to answer all of our questions. They responded with an enthusiastic "Yes!"

We got busy. DOT sent out an email blast to its staff, asking for volunteers who would be willing to work the first two or three Saturdays in August (the third Saturday was a "rain date" for the purposes of our evaluation). I did the same at the Department of Health and Mental Hygiene. By a week before the inaugural event, we'd trained our team of volunteers in data-collection methods. We gathered in a conference room at DOT's office, reviewed the data-collection forms, and answered questions. We went over what we would be doing at the event. On August 2—launch day—clipboards, pens, and clicker-counters were handed out. Last-minute preparations were made. We were ready to go.

Vicky Grimshaw and Sarah Wolf—the two staff members who had helped me get the Built Environment and Active Design Program off the ground—were on hand. We positioned ourselves at the three points where recreation stations had been set up—uptown, midtown, and downtown—and where crosstown traffic was being allowed by the New York Police Department. Along with our volunteers, we would be intercepting walkers, rollerbladers, and cyclists when they stopped at a traffic light. We'd ask them about their health status, their age, their home zip code, and their physical activity levels outside of the event, as well as the distances they'd traveled along the Summer Streets route.

The pilot evaluation on August 2 went well. But just as we had in West Virginia—my first experience with this type of "boots on the ground" work—we discovered that a few details of our procedure needed tweaking. It appeared we should stand on the side of the street where people were stopped at a red light, not on the other corner trying to stop them when they were already roaring forward on a green. If there were groups, we learned to survey all of them at once, or else the one person approached would likely say no to us and hurry to catch up with the others. And so we refined our methods and were ready to hit the streets again the following Saturday. I couldn't wait until the evaluations were complete and the results tabulated. I was so eager to learn what a program like Summer Streets could do to help get us moving.

The results were beyond encouraging. The fifty thousand people who took part in that inaugural event represented a healthy number for a new project. But I was even happier with the revelation that 87 percent of those who traveled to Summer Streets did so by walking, cycling, or taking public transport—all active modes of transportation. We also learned that about a quarter of those who attended were insufficiently active outside of Summer Streets. The event, then, was providing a much-needed opportunity for physical activity among those who didn't get enough in their daily lives. Score one for health. We also found that those who came out were getting about half of their weekly recommended physical activity at the event. In other words, Summer Streets was providing a significant opportunity to get physical activity, whether attendees chose to walk, cycle, rollerblade, or play. Chalk up another point for health. The outcomes that concerned the DOT—primarily, what impact the event would have on traffic congestion—were also positive: DOT assessments found no significant traffic delays created by the event!

I'd been a supporter of the Summer Streets idea from the moment I learned of it, and the evaluations we conducted that first August only heightened my enthusiasm. But having spent so much time "behind the scenes," I was eager to experience the event the way other New Yorkers did—by hitting the streets myself. And so the next year, and every year after, I set off on as many August Saturdays as I could, weather and schedule permitting.

In 2015, I enlisted other enthusiasts and made a trek through Summer Streets to the Brooklyn Bridge Park—one of several new green spaces opened during Mayor Bloomberg's administration. We'd been looking forward to this outing, and we weren't disappointed. On the wide sidewalks of South Harlem, we walked our bikes for the first five minutes to get from my apartment to Central Park. Then, entering the park at its north end, we hopped on and made the first strenuous uphill climb, slow and panting. The effort paid off, though, when we got to enjoy speeding downhill, wind against our faces, into the west side of the park and the Seventy-Second Street park road. We followed that road until we hit Park Avenue, where, even though it was only 8:00 a.m., the street was already jammed with "traffic": bikers, runners, rollerbladers, skateboarders, and walkers; men and women, boys and girls, parents with strollers. We passed people of all ages and races enjoying their Saturday morning with healthy, free activities. We rode quickly through intersections where the cross streets were barred by police, and stopped at red lights at the few large intersections that remained open. We gawked at the long lines of people waiting to be fitted for their new bicycle helmets being given out for free by DOT staff.

As we neared the Brooklyn Bridge, we stopped for a moment on the Manhattan side. Free drinking water was on offer from the New York City Department of Environmental Protection, which had hooked up their Water-on-the-Go fountains to hydrants. In Foley Square, flanked by the courthouses that viewers of *Law and Order* know so well, a "beach" had materialized out of thin air, complete with chairs, game stations, and a giant sixty-foot inflatable water slide. We stopped for a picture and a drink of water.

Then we were off again. We'd cycled about nine miles already, though it felt like nothing at all, with all the things to see along the way. We made our way onto the Brooklyn Bridge pedestrian and bicycle paths, following the cyclists in front of us in a single file and riding past the pedestrians on the right, many stopping for photographs of the Manhattan skyline or the Statue of Liberty in the distance.

Finally, Brooklyn. We made our way off the bridge, past a Citi Bike share station, and onto bicycle lanes on the quiet side streets of Brooklyn Heights. Finally, we arrived at Brooklyn Bridge Park. As we rode along New York's East River, with views of the newly finished Freedom Tower in front of us, we passed children's playgrounds, beach volleyball courts, a kayaking station, basketball courts, ball hockey play areas, and even exercise equipment, all free for public use. We were tempted to give a few a try, but we decided that our ride was enough for that day, and there were plenty of other people who wanted a turn. We stopped instead to grab a bite of lunch at a nearby restaurant—fuel for the ride back home. A perfect day.

Summer Streets is special—a limited opportunity to see and enjoy New York in a different way, during a typically warm month when people are looking for any excuse to get out and enjoy all that the city has to offer. But what about everyday needs? What about those kids we read about at the beginning of the chapter—the ones who have lost fine- and gross-motor skills because they head home and plant themselves on the couch after school rather than kicking a ball around with their neighbors?

A century ago, children used to play on the street: hide-and-seek until the streetlights came on; games of tag that lasted for hours; stickball and ball hockey; jump rope and hopscotch and hula hoops. They played baseball on the streets, to the consternation of neighbors whose house or apartment windows would sometimes be broken. Those days are largely gone, it would seem. Other, more sedentary activities—notably the lure of screens, or

perhaps the demands of excessive homework—seem to be imping-
ing on this active play time. Or maybe it's happening in a more
regimented, less spontaneous way, in the form of sports and organized activities for the children whose parents can afford the time
and money to involve their children in such. Additionally, outdoor space is often at a premium, and what little is available is
frequently given over to cars. In any case, what seems apparent
is that our kids are forgetting how to play—and becoming less
healthy in the process.

Perhaps my estimate of a century was optimistic. Maybe it's
been longer than that since kids could play safely on our city
streets. It was way back in 1914, after all, that New York's Police
Athletic League (PAL) created a program to make street play safe
for kids. At the time, there were more than thirty parks in
Manhattan, but very few were found in low-income neighborhoods. In a move designed to address that situation, Police
Commissioner Arthur Woods conducted a "play street" experiment. In July of that year, Eldridge Street between Rivington and
Delancey was closed to traffic. The Parks Department pitched in
with two street pianos, and the Eldridge Street Settlement organized a folk dance festival. All at once, a busy commercial block
had morphed into a place for play. The idea took off, and before
the end of the year, twenty-nine additional play streets could be
found around the city. By 1924, the program was operating in
the Bronx, Brooklyn, and Queens.

The idea behind Play Streets was simple: single blocks of city
streets would be closed to cars at certain hours of certain days
so that children could come out to play. The Police Athletic
League still runs Play Streets in New York in the summer months,
offering spaces for children to engage in both structured and
unstructured play. Programming exists to engage children, but
they are also free to ride their bicycles, practice their two- or
three-wheeled scootering, or just run around.

As wonderful as the PAL program was, it wasn't enough. By 2009, PAL funding for Play Streets was shrinking, and the number of Play Streets each summer was shrinking with it. It was a concern to those of us in the Built Environment and Active Design Program, and also to our new commissioner of Health, Tom Farley, who'd joined us when President Obama appointed Tom Frieden director of the CDC. Farley, formerly the dean of Public Health at Tulane University, had been working alongside his predecessor for about a year at the time and was familiar with the city's public health landscape. Not long after the changes took effect, Assistant Commissioner Lynn Silver passed along a message: our new commissioner wanted to see kids playing on the quieter streets of New York. "He's envisioning parents and neighbors sitting on their apartment stoops watching the kids play on the streets in front of their building," Lynn told me. "Can you make this happen?" I was certainly determined to try—and I knew exactly where to start.

For some time, the Department of Health and Mental Hygiene had been hearing from various community groups who were interested in hosting Play Streets of their own. For example, several farmers' markets thought it would be helpful to have Play Streets adjacent to their markets so that while the parents shopped for fruits and veggies, the children could play. What a perfect combination for health—if only we could find a way to give community groups the right to close off streets to cars and use them for children and families to play!

Our first call was to the Street Activity Permit Office, responsible largely for one-time events like neighborhood block parties. Sure, they said when we asked, community groups could apply for a Play Street event permit, "but only once a year."

Once a year? Children taking part in physical activity once a year was precisely the problem we were trying to remedy. We needed to find a way to allow children space to get physical activity on a much more regular basis: preferably multiple times each week or, best of all, daily. I turned next to my colleagues at the Department of Transportation. If we were talking about closing off streets, why not go directly to the source?

Andy Wiley-Schwartz had been an assistant commissioner hired by Janette Sadik-Khan, and he shared her commitment to creating vibrant public spaces in our cities. Andy came from the world of advocates, specifically a non-profit organization called Project for Public Spaces, which pushed for improvements to public spaces. Janette had put Andy in charge of the Plaza Program, and Andy was asking residents to propose new pedestrian spaces they wanted to see in their neighborhoods. I asked Andy if his staff could work with mine to set criteria for DOT approval of the closing of quieter streets to cars so children could use them for play at set days and times. He agreed to work with my team on a standardized application process—and gave his word that if the application was completed and the street and programming criteria were met, whether by a community group or a school, the Play Street would be approved.

And so, with DOT's help, the Play Streets program was expanded. Community groups like interested farmers' markets were now able to host Play Streets that PAL didn't have the capacity to run. And schools without enough play space for physical education or for active recess were also able to run Play Streets during set days and times on weekdays each week.

Play Streets was conceived of as an on-again, off-again program, but in some neighborhoods, Play Streets have become an everyday thing—an accomplishment that demonstrates just what can happen if a community comes together to fight for a common goal.

One evening during the summer of 2011, I attended a community board meeting in Jackson Heights. I was there to present information about the health benefits of physical activity—and physical activity spaces—for children. I was pleased to see that the meeting was well attended, with some parents even bringing along their five- and six-year-olds, some of whom were carrying banners asking for a place to play every day. Located in Queens, Jackson Heights is included on a list of areas in New York City's five boroughs with the least green space per capita. There was a playground in the neighborhood, but it was often overcrowded, and the adjacent street, although quiet, offered no help: children were not permitted to play there. The parents at the meeting wanted to access that additional space.

Thankfully, the community's voices were convincing, and so I was delighted to be able to return for the ribbon-cutting for the Jackson Heights Play Street. It was a hot summer day, and as we waited for some local politicians to arrive I took in the scene around me. Children and their parents gathered on the artificial turf laid in one corner of the street block where the children were playing with building blocks, unknowingly practicing their fine motor skills and burning calories as they stretched, stood up, and sat down again to stack the blocks. Kids stood in line, talking noisily as they waited their turn to climb inside the colorful bouncy castle, where each child was given time to jump on the air-filled nylon platform inside its netted space. Parents ran alongside children learning to ride small bicycles, or balancing on their two- or three-wheeled scooters and skateboards. Adults from the surrounding homes stood in small groups, chatting.

On August 13, 2011, *The New York Times* published an article by Alec Appelbaum entitled "Presto, Instant Playground." Likening Play Streets to today's trendy pop-up retail stores, Appelbaum described the initiative as pop-up playgrounds. In October of that same year, the *Chicago Tribune*'s Blair Kamin included Play Streets at number four in his "10 Steps to Begin Correcting Chicago's Open Space Shortage," citing New York City's efforts as an example for Chicago to follow.

Not long after, I spoke to Chicago's Department of Public Health about their desire to do just that. On a conference call, I discussed with them and their funder, Blue Cross Blue Shield of Illinois, how they could re-create Play Streets in their city. In 2012, the city launched PlayStreets Chicago. In the first year alone, the initiative attracted ten thousand attendees and hosted more than fifty events; by 2014, more than 140 events were organized. Sixty-four percent of attendees reported that they would have engaged in sedentary activity had it not been for the PlayStreets—a number that matched our findings in New York, where the majority of parents surveyed on site reported that their children would have been inside or watching television had the Play Street not been available. Evaluations at these Play Street sites showed that children were staying at Play Streets for between an hour and two and a half hours, on average.

As with so many successful initiatives, this one took a combination of need (a safe place for children to play), inspiration (a great idea that was being underutilized), and cooperation (between various government departments and community groups) to come to fruition. A generation of children in Jackson Heights, in Chicago, and beyond will be happier, and healthier, for the effort.

Move to Improve

In addition to play space creation in and around schools and neighborhoods, which was the purview of the Built Environment and Active Design Program, the Department of Health and Mental Hygiene wanted to make sure our schools were following through on healthy activity initiatives within their own walls.

While working with New York's bodegas to increase healthy food offerings in some of the city's highest-needs neighborhoods (see chapter 2), the Physical Activity and Nutrition Program initiated by Candace Young and her deputy, Sabrina Baronberg, also created a program that would eventually come to be called Move to Improve. Early on, Candace found state funding that could be utilized to provide daycares and schools with health programming assistance. As she and her staff plowed through the scientific literature, looking for programs they could adopt, SPARK and CATCH both caught their eye. Called "a school-based solution to our nation's healthcare crisis" in the Surgeon General's Report, SPARK is designed to get children more active during their school days. It provides a curriculum package—complete with training, follow-up support, and equipment—to teachers and recreation leaders serving the pre-kindergarten through grade twelve community. For example, CDs and simple equipment like satin ribbons might be provided to teachers to "spark" physical activity even within limited classroom spaces. Peek in during one of these sessions and you might see kids following along after their teacher, moving their arms up and down to music as their little hands grip the flowing ribbons. Some might be giggling and having a good time, while others might be concentrating hard, and slightly flushed from the physical exertion.

CATCH—which stands for Coordinated Approach to Child Health—takes a wider approach by aiming to help children make healthy food choices and increase the amount of physical activity they get each day. Consider a community baseball game. Jose's up to bat, and he gets a hit! In a CATCH program, all of the children, rather than Jose alone, would run the bases.

Candace was intrigued by these programs and the possibilities they presented. Initially, she'd use the funding she'd found to create a training program for daycare workers and elementary school teachers in SPARK—and later Move to Improve (a very similar program adapted from SPARK)—and to purchase the necessary CDs and accompanying activity supplies. Evaluations would eventually find that the Move to Improve program introduced into daycares and elementary schools in New York would add an average of twelve minutes of physical activity to each school day, an hour more activity to the school week.

Participation Marks

Summer Streets, Play Streets, Move to Improve—I was so excited to see these programs up and running, and growing in popularity. They were important weapons in the battle we were waging against obesity and its many consequences. And they had all, in various ways, proven just how effective alliances between different government departments and with non-government entities could be. Community groups, non-profits, corporations: all had roles to play. That realization got those of us in the Built Environment and Active Design Program at the health department thinking about what other innovative partnerships could be created for the expansion of healthy opportunities and options. As Sarah Wolf and I brainstormed, we kept coming back to a group that we hadn't yet consulted: students. Could we somehow partner with students themselves? Could students—particularly high schoolers, but even middle schoolers—be engaged in helping us identify and make changes within their schools or communities to support a more healthy lifestyle?

It's 4:00 p.m. on a school day, and I am making my way to the YMCA in Long Island City, Queens. It has been a year or so since the Active Design Guidelines were published, and Sarah Wolf, who assisted me in writing the first chapter on health and the built environment, and in corralling our various partners to write their pieces too, has made a transition from Built Environment Coordinator to Community Engagement Coordinator for our Built Environment and Active Design Program. Like the rest of our program's team, Sarah was still responsible for Active Design in New York City, but her work now focused on the public engagement aspects. The day is gray and chilly, and

I'm wearing a down coat, hat, and gloves as I walk across the bridge from my office—recently relocated from downtown Manhattan—over the train tracks to the other side, where LaGuardia Community College and the YMCA are located. As I enter the building through automatic sliding doors that open as I approach, I revel in the warmth. The woman at the front desk directs me to a room down the hallway to the right. I open the door and inch my way in.

Sarah waves to me from the far side of the room by the windows, where she is sitting at one of the student desks that have been arranged in a large circle. The desks are filled with middle school students who are participating in this YMCA after-school program on civic engagement. I've arrived just in time to hear the student presentations—a practice session for the real presentations they'll be giving, along with students from other YMCAs, to public officials who have volunteered for a student civic engagement event that's coming up soon.

This particular YMCA after-school program is brainstorming and identifying improvements that could be made to the surrounding neighborhood to improve health. Early on, Sarah had spoken to the students about the epidemics of obesity and diabetes in the United States and in New York in particular, and about the evidence for addressing physical activity and healthier diets through interventions to the built environment, including those for improving active transportation, active recreation, active buildings, and actively promoting healthy food and beverage access. Over the years, these four components have become the pillars of our work in the Built Environment and Active Design Program of New York City's Department of Health and Mental Hygiene. Now, these students are applying this knowledge.

Several groups have decided to take on active transportation, and the first has chosen to consider the intersection just outside this YMCA. It features a crisscross pattern of diagonal crosswalks, with a triangle of unmarked space in the center that neither cars nor pedestrians can use. "We would like to make a pedestrian plaza here," says a presenter, a girl of about thirteen, with long dark hair, jeans, and black sneakers with neon pink laces, who is wearing her short ski jacket even though we are inside the warm classroom. An earlier presenter has already cited the dangers of the intersection, along with accident statistics. She goes on to describe the features of the pedestrian plaza they have in mind: "Chairs and tables, pots of plants to put around the plaza, a painted floor to make it visible." A third presenter takes over and lists the various groups they'd need to try to engage in order to create the plaza.

I am so impressed by these young men and women. Not only have they taken in what Sarah has told them about our work, but they've also applied it to their own lives and experiences in a meaningful way. I leave the meeting that day feeling inspired and hopeful; if we can get the next generation of activists, architects, doctors, lawyers, and government leaders on board at such an early age, how can we not succeed in changing our cities—and our health outcomes—for the better?

Over the next few years Sarah would invite me to see similar presentations by other youth. One came from high school students whose teachers worked with the Built Environment and Active Design Program to integrate our content on active transportation, active buildings, active recreation, and actively increasing access to healthy foods and beverages—in other words, Active Design—into their classes. This classroom brainstorming would eventually lead to successes such as those taking place in Harlem.

Harlem, New York, is a neighborhood in transition. Two decades ago, it was a dangerous spot, best avoided by anyone who didn't live there. Today, Harlem is a hip and diverse place to live, with young singles and young families moving in in recent years. New cafés and their bustling patios pop up practically weekly, and celebrity chefs like Marcus Samuelsson, born in Ethiopia and raised in Scandinavia, are opening more and more trendy restaurants that attract local and international foodies alike.

Harlem is also home to Innovation High School—an educational facility that clearly highlights the important role students themselves can play when it comes to improving their schools. Through implementing workshops there that Sarah and I had previously created for youth and community residents, the students identified elements in the physical environment that presented barriers to healthy lifestyles: difficulties accessing stairways, for example, or a lack of access to drinking water. This in itself is great news—awareness is half the battle—but in Innovation High School, the students took things a step further by actively engaging in making the physical changes happen. They painted and installed murals on their stairwell walls, making the stairs an inviting space. They advocated for funding for new water fountains, and then decorated the spaces around them. And they created point-of-decision messages to remind their classmates to undertake healthy behaviors, like choosing water over a sugary drink. Evaluations conducted by my team and our partners in the initiative, including Mount Sinai Hospital, showed that healthy behaviors increased after the interventions.

As the kids themselves had correctly identified in our workshops, the environments outside their schools were also critical in terms of impacting their health. Did the sidewalks in the neighborhood make it possible to walk safely to and from school? Were there options for biking? What food sources could be found in the surrounding neighborhood? While the students have learned to look for and identify issues like these, they are aware that they have less agency outside their school walls. They need help, from community organizations and others who can think creatively about ways to get us all moving.

Playful Cities

I met Dr. William Bird for the first time in 2009, at New York City's Walk21 Conference—an international conference devoted to walking and achieving livable, sustainable cities—where he was giving a keynote speech on health. His "day job" is as a family physician in London, but in spite of his trademark conservative suit, plain white shirt, and dark tie, William is no ordinary clinician. In addition to seeing patients, he is also the founder of Intelligent Health, a company dedicated to promoting physical activity. William is particularly interested in promoting walking. In fact, the company has an initiative—called Beat the Street— that turns walking into a bit of competitive fun. Working in tandem with a city's transportation department, the company supplies devices that can be installed on street signs and other street structures. Working solo or in teams, participants pick up a Beat the Street card, which contains radio-frequency identification (RFID) technology, and then taps it against sensors called Beat Boxes when they are out and about. They receive points for each box they tap, and prizes for tapping the most boxes. The end result: schools, community groups, and businesses get motivated, and an entire community gets more active. In 2016, more than two hundred thousand people engaged in the program in the U.K. and beyond, and 78 percent reported becoming more active.

Programs like Beat the Street are particularly intriguing when it comes to enticing more children to walk to school—and for parents to let them. In 2005, a report from the CDC stated that only 15 percent of children in the United States walk to school. This contrasts with the 50 percent who walked to school in 1969 (a figure that rose to 87 percent for those living within a mile from the school). According to the CDC report, the barriers most commonly cited by parents with children aged five to eighteen years old were distance, traffic dangers, and weather. Weather clearly hasn't changed significantly since 1969, but we are certainly building larger schools to serve larger areas, which increases walking distance. And wider roads designed for more and faster cars are also a modern trend.

William's company is well aware of these dangers. And so, his scanning devices are installed on safe walking routes that have been mapped out for the schoolchildren. In some of his pilot sites in the U.K., "walking school buses" were created. These adult-supervised walks to and from school along safe routes have been tried and studied in other communities around the globe, including in North America, reassuring parents. With Beat the Street, everyone wins.

William Bird is certainly not alone in his goal of making physical activity fun and of getting cities involved. In November 2013, I traveled to San Francisco to attend the Design Like You Give a Damn conference, organized by Architecture for Humanity. Before it filed for bankruptcy in 2015, Architecture for Humanity was a Bay Area non-profit whose mission was to find architectural solutions to humanitarian issues globally. I had been invited to moderate a panel on Design and Health, which is where I met fellow panel member Darell Hammond. Darell spoke passionately about the importance of play for children—and for adults. He spoke about the loss of play within our society and our lives. He spoke about bringing play back. It was a pleasure to listen to him speak so passionately about a topic of shared interest.

Darell's quiet manner can be deceptive; it belies a determination that has convinced many corporations to donate significant sums of money. When he's not speaking at conferences, Darell is the CEO and founder of KaBOOM!, a non-profit organization that helps build playgrounds. Using a participatory design process, KaBOOM! elicits input from the community and even erects their playgrounds with the help of community members. One success story involves a community of just a few thousand people that was coping with several teen suicides every year. With funding in hand from their corporate donors, KaBOOM! got to work, making sure they engaged the community's teens in the building process. In the year after the playground was constructed, there were no additional teen suicides. It's a situation, I'm told, that the organization continues to monitor. Sometimes, play can be about much more than physical health.

I'd known about KaBOOM! for a few years by the time Darell and I met in person, but we hadn't had yet found a way to work together. That changed a few months after the San Francisco conference, when I received an email from James Siegal, KaBOOM!'s chief administrative officer. He was going to be in New York City. Could we meet? Over iced lattes in Times Square on a hot summer afternoon, James got straight to the point: Would I like to take part in a summit that KaBOOM! would be hosting that fall?

As adults, few of us expect to attend work conferences on play—and yet, that's exactly what KaBOOM!'s event turned out to be. In late October 2014—after several months of advisory discussions with KaBOOM!—I touched down in Chicago for the Playful Cities USA Conference. The next day, KaBOOM! staff dressed in purple and orange T-shirts greeted the organizers, advisers, and participants outside the venue, which was festooned with purple and orange balloons. They ushered us into a conference room, where chairs had been set up as usual at large, round tables. But there were signs that this conference was going to be something out of the ordinary: six-foot-tall "palm trees" lined the walls of the room, made out of more purple and orange balloons.

Darell stood on the stage at the front of the room. Once everyone was seated and the lights were dimmed, he began his welcome. Next, the CEO of Humana, the health insurance company that was sponsoring the conference, made his remarks. Soon enough, we were on to the highlight of the event. The attending cities, twelve in all, were there to share their play-related projects with one another, and to get advice from the panel of advisers (myself included). The idea was to talk about creating more playful cities in the United States. Over the course of the next several hours, we heard from Bloomington, Indiana; Brownsville, Texas; Chicago, Illinois; Durham, North Carolina; Memphis, Tennessee; Ottawa, Kansas; Pittsburgh, Pennsylvania; Providence, Rhode Island; San Francisco, California; Spartanburg, South Carolina; Washington, D.C.; and York, Pennsylvania.

It turned out, though, that Playful Cities USA was not the only conference dedicated to play. In fact, there is an International Play Association (IPA), and even a Triennial International Play Association Conference, which has convened nineteen times, to date. The IPA was formed more than fifty years ago in Denmark as the International Association for the Child's Right to Play. Since then, more than forty countries have signed on to support the 1959 United Nations Declaration of the Rights of the Child, which includes the statement: "the child shall have full opportunity for play and recreation which should be directed to the same purposes as education."

In 1989, the General Assembly of the United Nations affirmed these rights in its Convention on the Rights of the Child—"the right to rest and leisure, to engage in play and recreational activities, appropriate for the age of the child"—in addition to the rights to a name, nationality, health care services, education, protection against discrimination, protection against abuse/neglect/injury, and protection against economic exploitation.

In May 2014, the 19th International Play Association Conference was held in Istanbul, Turkey, and focused on the reasons for play, play spaces, and play and the media. In 2017, Calgary, Alberta, hosted the twentieth conference.

I learned that Calgary would be hosting the 2017 conference back in 2013, when I attended a roundtable there hosted by

Vivo, a local recreation center whose vision and work has transcended its physical boundaries. Once known as Cardel Place, the center was renamed to allude to the life and living that can be fostered by play, recreation, and physical activity. Since 2013, Vivo has held two such roundtables to promote play and active recreation, both within its own walls and outside of them.

At that first gathering, Vivo had rallied a range of stakeholders— recreation department staff, non-profit organization representatives, and key political figures, including then premier Jim Prentice—to speak. In a keynote presentation, I shared my work with other cities and the lessons that could be learned around physical activity and play. The roughly two hundred participants actively discussed the state of play in Calgary and in the province of Alberta, and brainstormed the next steps needed to promote improvements in the paltry levels of physical activity seen in children and adults. Participants identified who was there and who was missing. Although many recreation professionals were present, it became clear after my keynote that there were others who needed to be engaged—planners, for example, and transportation professionals, without whom recreation and play facilities may remain less accessible for large numbers of children and adults. Calgary was off to a great start. In 2015, Vivo would host its second roundtable, again with its key partners the City of Calgary and Mount Royal University.

But Vivo's commitment goes beyond dialogue. In the days following the first roundtable, Vivo asked me to meet with the architecture team from the design firm (aptly called Dialog) that was helping with their recreation center expansions. Vivo emphasized the need and desire for greater influence in the neighborhood and community. I suggested a model that would take them into the community as well as bring community members into their facility. We discussed such concepts as permeability and transparency of space and programming, where the community flowed into Vivo's space and Vivo's staff and programs flowed, in turn, into the community.

This idea of permeability is taking hold more and more, with greater efforts to bring play and activity programming outside the walls of formal recreation organizations. South of the Canadian border, the U.S. Centers for Disease Control and Prevention has provided funding to entities like the YMCA to stretch their play and recreation programs beyond their walls and into communities, particularly to try to connect with hard-to-reach populations, including the many people who have no desire to go to a gym. Other cities have taken a less formal approach, relying on programming delivered in a more ad hoc way, by residents.

The persistent buzz of the alarm pulls me from sleep. Groggy and disoriented, I squint at the clock: 4:00 a.m. A knock on my door startles me and I sit bolt upright and look around. It's my second day in Taipei, and clearly, the jetlag hasn't worn off quite yet. I call out to Radha Chaddah, on the other side of the hotel room door, that I will be ready for breakfast in fifteen minutes. I rush to put on my jeans and T-shirt and throw on a sweatshirt to protect me against the morning chill. I head to Radha's room, where we both wolf down our room-service breakfast of eggs and fruit.

Radha and I are in Taiwan's capital city because of a conversation we had several months earlier in Shanghai. Radha is in her mid-forties, a medical doctor, lawyer, and public health professional by training. We became friends in New York. She moved to Taipei, briefly, before relocating to Shanghai, where she and her husband now make their home. During her time in Taipei, Radha observed a phenomenon that aroused her insatiable curiosity— the use of public parks by seniors. During our Shanghai visit, after a morning tour of the newly renovated Bund walking path, Radha wondered if we could study the seniors in Taipei. "It's amazing how they swarm the public parks every morning," she said. "From my window, I could see every corner of the park across from our apartment filled with seniors exercising. Every day."

Less than a year later and here we are. After Radha had proposed the idea, I started to look for funding. I'd been recently appointed an adjunct professor of the newly formed School of Public Health at the University of Alberta. A longtime colleague mentioned that he had some leftover funding. Dr. Don Schopflocher is a biostatistician who worked for many years with the Alberta Ministry of Health; he'd been my co-chair for a provincial chronic disease risk factor surveillance working group during my years as deputy medical officer in Edmonton, prior to my move to Atlanta. At the same time, Sylvie Stachenko, the new dean of Public Health at the University of Alberta, had asked me to assist her in the advancement of global initiatives for chronic disease prevention. Sylvie's wish, Radha's idea, and Don's funding came together perfectly. If we could understand the phenomenon in Taipei, we reasoned, perhaps we could apply the lessons learned to promoting more play among the seniors in North America, too.

After our quick breakfast, Radha and I make our way to the lobby to meet Irene—our guide, translator, photographer, and videographer. It's still dark outside when we climb into Irene's car for the short drive to a nearby public park. We arrive a little before 5:00 a.m. The sun has only just begun to rise, but we can see from the pink and orange hues in the sky that it's going to be a beautiful, sunny day. Radha and I clamber out of Irene's hatchback. The early morning air is chilly; dewdrops still cling to the roofs of the cars parked overnight nearby.

From the park entrance we see that the space is already filling up. Men and women—elderly but agile—are everywhere. On the paths around the rim of the park we see some joggers, but mostly walkers. We wait for several seniors on bikes to ride past, conversing with each other while riding at a leisurely pace. As we cross the path and enter the park, we notice a large group to our right.

Music plays as the paired men and women sway back and forth. Ballroom dancing. To our left is a playground, where seniors are using the equipment. One lifts his right leg onto a step leading up to the slide and leans into a stretch. Another hoists herself onto the monkey bars, swings her legs up and over, and drops from the bar to hang upside down. "Good for circulation," a senior walking by tells Irene, who translates for me.

The number of seniors stretching and hanging off the children's playground equipment is stunning. And straight ahead of us are even more. A large group of women move in step with each other as they follow a leader in the moves of a traditional Chinese dance. Next to them, another group of men and women lift their arms in unison in *qi gong* exercises to improve the circulation of their *qi*, or energy. Another group is two-stepping to country music, some with cowboy hats on. In the distance, seniors are playing Frisbee. It isn't easy to make our way across the park through the crowds. Chinese dancing, western dancing, ballroom dancing, aerobics, tai chi, Frisbee, badminton, ball playing, walking, running, karaoke—groups stretch across the park lawn for as far as I can see.

After that first eye-opening morning, we settled into a regular routine. Irene would head off to take photographs and record video footage to document the incredible phenomena we were witnessing between 4:30 and 10:00 a.m. daily. Radha and I would use a data collection instrument called SOPARC to capture user counts and activity levels. We would each mark our observations on our own SOPARC forms and then compare them later. And when Irene was ready to translate, we would approach seniors and ask if we could interview them about their use of the park.

We visited five parks during our week in the city. We learned that seniors use the parks daily or nearly daily. They come to exercise but, just as important, to meet their friends. Most live near the park, although some travel by bus from farther away. Almost all said they felt safe, even at 4:00 a.m. when the sky was still dark. It was easy to see why. The presence of so many eyes in the park—watching from exercise groups, from their walks, from their bikes; watching upside down from the monkey bars—helped to ensure that unsavory activities didn't occur. The group instructors (also seniors) told us they volunteered to lead the classes. They had a skill and time on their hands, they said, so why not share it with others? Why not contribute to their neighborhoods and communities? Those who took the classes often donated money to help the instructors pay for music CDs and boombox batteries, and the instructors told us they got a free permit from Taipei's parks department to teach their classes. We asked if it was hard to get the permit. Not at all, they would reply. "We apply, and three days later we get the permit."

Back in our hotel, poring over the day's photos and footage, Radha and I would compare what we'd seen to the situation in North America, where so many seniors are isolated, forced into dependency on others by stiffening bones and joints exacerbated by the lack of movement and play, and, in many cases, by the lack of opportunities to move anywhere without a car. Even those who might live within walking distance of a park find themselves at a loss for company in these facilities that are too often empty of people on weekdays. Play is not a part of their lives. We'd ask ourselves: What can we learn from Taipei? How can we bring more play into the lives of adults, and particularly seniors, in North American cities?

Seven years have passed since our study in Taipei. Our paper was published in 2014, along with a YouTube video entitled *Understanding Older Adults' Use of Green Spaces in Taipei, Taiwan*, put together from Irene's footage. The response has been encouraging. Parks and recreation departments across North America have joined the discussion, asking how we can bring more play into the lives of adults, children, and seniors.

Creating Space for Play

My visit to Taipei underlined something I'd known for a long time: while it's absolutely wonderful to give children and families an opportunity to play safely on city streets, and to ensure that physical activity is a part of the day from the earliest years right on through to adulthood, progress on that front doesn't negate the need for open spaces, green spaces, and dedicated play spaces in our cities. In 2010 developer Jonathan Rose described to Fit City 5 attendees the ideal developments for people and the environment. What we should strive to achieve, he said, is "density with green spaces, density with spaces for respite." With density, achieved by mixing a variety of housing types, comes a sufficient number of people to make amenities nearby such as stores, schools, and parks possible and affordable. That's a good thing. But density is also . . . crowded. All of those people whose purchasing power and taxes support amenities can be a bit much at times, and we can find ourselves needing a break. That's where space for play—in one form or another—comes in.

But in cities like New York—ones that are very nearly fully built, with boundaries that prevent further geographic area growth— building such spaces is not always an easy feat. An important driver of the innovations for open spaces, green spaces, and play spaces in New York City has been PlaNYC 2030—the same plan that helped to drive the expansion of bicycling infrastructure, pedestrian amenities, and Bus Rapid Transit. On the green space front, the stated goal was for every New Yorker to live within a ten-minute walk of a park or playground. Areas without space for new parks and playgrounds—and where residents lacked access to them within a ten-minute walk—would be targeted for new parks through renovations of and community access to school-yards, or through the creation of pedestrian plazas that could function as pocket parks. The expansion of the Play Streets pro-grams was introduced as one way to reach the "ten-minute access" goal. In 2011, an updated version of PlaNYC was released. With the work I had been coordinating across different New York City agencies, we were able to integrate public health as a PlaNYC goal in and of itself (as opposed to a pleasant offshoot of other goals).

With PlaNYC offering a roadmap of sorts, the Department of Parks and Recreation has been working with organizations such as the Trust for Public Land to convert schoolyards into community playgrounds. Since 1996, more than 180 playgrounds have been built in New York City schools by this partnership, adding up to 150 additional acres of play space serving 4.5 million additional residents. The spaces are used by the school during school hours and remain open for community use during non-school hours and on weekends. Community participation has been a vital part of the process, with input from school staff, students, parents, and residents gathered during three months of participatory design. The resulting spaces have transformed barren asphalt into brightly painted track facilities, with athletic and play amenities and equipment desired by students and nearby residents.

The parks department has been busy in other ways as well. An initiative that began during Mayor Michael Bloomberg's administration and continues today has seen more than 850 acres of new parkland added to the city, much of it along the waterfront. New recreational facilities were opened in all five boroughs. New York City beaches have become more accessible, with mats placed on the sand to allow those in wheelchairs to move themselves to the water's edge. And residents and tourists alike can now bicycle, rollerblade, run, or walk nearly the entire length of the west side of Manhattan alongside the Hudson River on a greenway protected from car traffic. The hope, moving forward, is to encircle Manhattan in a continuous greenway loop that features a variety of amenities: tennis courts, basketball courts, art installations, free kayaking, restaurants, and water fountains.

———

To attract users of different types, with different interests and different needs, a variety of types of parks and play spaces is important. So, in addition to community playgrounds and large parks with facilities for team or individual sports, it's great to have parks for walking or bicycling to and then simply hanging out. One of the crowning achievements of Bloomberg's administration was the creation of just such a space: the now world-renowned High Line Park.

Perched above the city streetscape on the west side of lower Manhattan, and in part inspired by Paris's Promenade Plantée, the High Line is a walking park that opened in June 2009. It's a wonderful space, nearly 1.5 miles of a linear path that takes you under buildings, through ever-changing art installations next to the path and sometimes painted or projected onto housing and commercial buildings that abut the pathway, through landscapes and skylines; a view of the Empire State Building is available from one angle, and the distant Statue of Liberty can be seen from another. You can walk through grassier areas, areas with more vegetation and trees, areas with more buildings around you, areas with water features where you can remove your shoes and dip your feet in summer, areas with drinking fountains that also water the plants around you, areas with benches made from the wood of the old railroad tracks and placed right onto the metal tracks left behind on the path. There are amphitheater-style seats with a rectangular frame suggesting a screening you should watch, but in place of a screen, you see the street life of the city below and in front of you. And it all sits, believe it or not, on abandoned elevated railway tracks.

Opened in 1934, after street-level tracks were deemed to be causing too many accidents, the elevated High Line tracks connected freight trains directly to factories and warehouses. Raw and manufactured goods, as well as meat, produce, and dairy products, could be transported and unloaded without disturbing street traffic. For a time, the practice was revolutionary, but as truck transport increased throughout the United States, rail traffic dropped, and after the last train rumbled through in 1980, the tracks fell into disrepair. Demolitions were petitioned for and expected, but in 1999, two friends, Joshua David and Robert Hammond, discovered the abandoned tracks and decided a different outcome was possible. They founded the conservancy organization called Friends of the High Line, and soon after, pictures of the abandoned tracks began to surface—overgrown with native grasses and weeds, but with the beautiful New York skyline above, and the Hudson River just to the west. It didn't take long for the movement to save the High Line to gain momentum.

Soon after Mayor Bloomberg was elected, Amanda Burden was appointed commissioner of New York City's Department of City Planning. Amanda quickly became a Friend of the High Line, and along with the conservancy founders, began to envision a new amenity for the far west side of the Chelsea neighborhood. They pictured a world-class park perched above the city's streets, with vistas of the Hudson River and views of New York's greatest landmarks, from the Statue of Liberty to the Empire State Building. With Amanda's urging and support, the City of New York got on board.

The process wasn't easy. Complex and creative zoning methods were used to compensate the developers who'd purchased the property below the tracks with an eye toward developing it following demolition. The City transferred the property rights to other available City-owned lands, nearby but away from the tracks. Though the Friends of the High Line worked hard to raise money, the City of New York also invested dollars—in the nine-figure range—into the redevelopment project.

In 2006, breaking ground for the tracks' conversion began with landscape architecture firm Diller Scofidio + Renfro and planting designer Piet Oudolf. The parks department's Charles

McKinney and I worked with Claire Weisz of WXY Studio to design and place new and innovative health- and environment-enhancing elements within the park space (including those innovative water fountains without drains described in chapter 2). Users would never have to shy away from drinking zero-calorie healthy tap water from a clogged fountain, and the water draining off the front of the fountain would run into the ground to quench the surrounding plants. Since the High Line's opening, residential and commercial real estate development and retail business around the park has boomed. The City has recouped its investment dollars many times over to the tune of billions, and now, with Phase 2 opened in 2011 and the third and final phase opened in 2014, both financial returns as well as users of the park continue to soar. As of July 2014, over twenty million people had visited the High Line.

The use of old railway tracks and unused and abandoned lands to create rejuvenated spaces is not unique to New York City. Many other cities have embraced rails-to-trails projects. In the United States, a national non-profit organization, the Rails-to-Trails Conservancy, based in Washington, D.C., is working to create a network of trails on unused tracks across the country.

My old haunt, Atlanta—home of the Centers for Disease Control and Prevention, and the birthplace of this work for me—has also been busy on this front. The Atlanta Beltline is a greenway trail being developed from a twenty-two-mile abandoned railway track encircling downtown Atlanta. The development is far-ranging and includes considerations for transit connections, housing (including affordable housing), and green space, as well as a greenway that connects forty-five different neighborhoods in town. It was conceived in 1999 by Georgia Institute of Technology student Ryan Gravel as the work of his master's thesis. Though far from a done deal (2030 is the anticipated date of completion), four sections of the Beltline and six new or renovated parks are now open.

And then there's Seoul, Korea. The Cheonggyecheon area in downtown Seoul was named after a stream, though until recently you'd have been hard-pressed to figure out why. For many years, that beautiful stream—which had once run near several historical palaces—was covered by a highway. In 2003, Mayor Lee Myung-bak began a massive undertaking to remove the fifty-foot-wide highway built in 1976, and to pump 120,000 tons of water back into the dried-up streambed. The huge undertaking was part of an effort to revitalize the downtown economy, to restore the area's connections to Korean culture and history, and to introduce greenery into a concrete urban jungle.

In 2006, the newly restored stream and a series of pedestrian paths were opened to the public to great acclaim and delight. But this wasn't the only good news associated with the project. As Mayor Myung-bak had hoped, there were environmental and economic benefits as well. Temperatures in nearby areas, which had previously been heat islands due to all the concrete and steel, cooled to healthier levels. Cheonggyecheon is now listed as one of the major tourist attractions in Seoul. Within a decade, it had become a cultural and economic center for the city—proving once again that public health and economic health need not be mutually exclusive, and that all of our cities have something to gain by embracing play.

Sharing Knowledge

The topic of play was front and center at the 2013 Active Living Research (ALR) Conference in sunny San Diego. That's where I met Suzanne Davies, who was working with Nike on their Designed to Move project. Nike had created Designed to Move as a vehicle for working with partners to promote physical activity. At the time, they were deep into the first component: Active Schools.

They were, however, interested in a second component: Active Cities. At the ALR Conference, Suzanne heard all about the growing research showing the strong links between how we design our cities, buildings, streets, neighborhoods, and their amenities, and physical activity levels in our children, adults, and seniors.

Soon after Suzanne returned to Portland, Oregon, where Nike was headquartered, she asked me to take part in a conference call with some of her staff. Designed to Move wanted to use the available evidence on the built environment and physical activity to transform cities around the world. Nike certainly knew how to do marketing. So, how could we combine those marketing skills, the available evidence being generated by researchers around the world, and my experience helping municipal governments to make more cities more active?

Together we would embark on a journey, along with other partners, to create *Active Cities: A Guide for City Leaders*. Designed to Move began by convening a group of experts in New York City in the fall of 2013. Researchers from the United States, Brazil, China, and beyond took part, along with non-profit organizations focused on play, like KaBOOM! and the Trust for Public Land. Dr. Jim Sallis of Active Living Research and I were asked to facilitate discussions that would summarize both the research and the processes and strategies for action. During a break, I intercepted Jim at the coffee station. Something was on my mind. Why stop at physical activity outcomes? I wondered. Wouldn't it be helpful to policy-makers, like the ones I worked with in cities around the world, to know about the other outcomes that could result from interventions to improve our buildings, streets, and neighborhoods for physical activity? Outcomes related to the environment and the economy, for example? I told Jim that I'd encountered a few studies on the topic, but nothing more. "To have all of this summarized in one place would be amazing," I said. Jim agreed.

Published in 2015, *Active Cities* did just that: in the very first section of the guide, we summarized the multiple outcomes and benefits cities could reap if they designed their environments to promote physical activity. The paper I'd released—along with the team from the Johns Hopkins Center for Injury Research and Policy and the Society for Public Health Education—had already demonstrated the overlap of strategies for physical activity and injury prevention. Now we'd have a document that showed a host of other important benefits to community leaders.

The guide's second section showed city leaders what to do— step by step. In my experiences across multiple cities, key actions had emerged. First was to prioritize physical activity by creating visible leadership on the issue; integrating physical activity directly into the goals of a city's master plan and guiding documents; and aligning city departments on the issue. Next, city leaders needed to think about making existing resources in their city active resources. All cities have streets, so it would be important to ensure that these streets accommodated active transportation modes such as walking, cycling, and transit, not only sedentary ones like the car. And since all cities have buildings, ensuring that physical activity opportunities are built into the building's amenities for occupants, such as the ability to use pleasant and safe stairs, would be crucial. Active play resources could be made even more accessible and safe: schools could open up their playgrounds and play spaces for the community to use after hours; play amenities could be lit at night to extend the hours of play.

It was also crucial for city leaders to design for people to be active. To do that, city leaders needed to find out what their residents wanted and to design for them; they needed to ensure everyone would be included, especially those most vulnerable to inactivity, such as those who might have disabilities, the elderly, and teenage girls, among others. Affordable access also must be considered and improved for those whose incomes may make it challenging to access costly recreation programs and facilities. And physical activity considerations had to be integrated into all city policies. Finally, city leaders needed to create a legacy of physical activity by activating public demand for it, and by leaving behind lasting infrastructures and policies that would promote physical activity.

The group that met in New York in the fall of 2013 to discuss *Active Cities* had also recommended including case studies from around the world. To keep the guide from getting too big, it was decided that ten case studies would be used, reflecting cities of different sizes and cultures: Hernando, Mississippi (population 15,000); Buenos Aires, Argentina (population 3 million); New York, New York (population 8.2 million); Copenhagen, Denmark (population 2 million); Rio de Janeiro, Brazil (population 12 million); Medellin, Colombia (population 3.7 million); Red Deer, Canada (population 100,000); Bristol, U.K. (population 437,000); and Adelaide, Australia (city population 22,200; state population 1,685,700).

The range of sizes and types of cities was a testament to the progress feasible across the globe. In Hernando, Mississippi, with a population of 15,000, there were many streets that were wider than necessary, and the city used the opportunity to paint bicycle lanes on them. Highway underpasses, previously used to move cattle in the 1960s, were repurposed into safe pedestrian and cyclist crossings. Empty pastures were transformed into fields for youth soccer programs. Medellin, Colombia, a city of nearly 4 million residents, was featured for its public parks with free exercise equipment as well as its cable-car system created to connect people without access to other transportation to public parks and even to jobs. Red Deer, Canada, with its approximately 100,000 people, was featured for its new sidewalk-clearing policy standard, as well as for making better connections between recreational paths and on-street bicycle lanes and better connections between transit stops and sidewalks and trails.

One of my favourite parts of *Active Cities*, though, is likely something few others would even notice. In the last few pages of the guide—after the resource section and several pages of citations—is an impressive list of key contributors and participants. The National League of Cities in the United States is there, along with the Urban Planning Society of China and EMBARQ Brasil, an organization dedicated to improving urban planning and transportation issues in Brazilian cities. The United Nations Development Program, which helps to build cities in under-resourced countries, is also noted. Even now, a few years after the guide's publication, I smile when I look at this page. To me, this list represents support and buy-in. It represents like-minded organizations, cities, and governments. It's an enormously satisfying list for someone who has devoted her career to exploring the links between how we build and design our cities and our health. These organizations and governments—these people— are allies in the fight to use much-needed interventions to improve our health outcomes.

9 | SPREADING THE WORD

BRINGING FIT CITY CONCEPTS TO THE WORLD

THE WORLD IS waking up to the fact that cities need to support people who want to be more healthy and live healthier lifestyles by making sure that options for healthy living exist—whether in terms of food choices, building choices, or transportation and recreation choices.

In 2013, I had been running the Built Environment Program (to which "Active Design" was added once we published those guidelines in 2010) in New York for seven years. It was satisfying work—work that I loved—but as the Active Design and Fit City movements picked up steam, consulting requests were coming in from all over the world: the Heart and Stroke Foundation of Canada; the Australian Heart Foundation; the Premier's Council for Active Living in New South Wales, Australia; Peel Region in Ontario, Canada; the Office of the Chief Medical Officer of Health in Alberta, Canada; the School of Public Health and the School of Urban and Regional Planning at the University of Alberta; the Shanghai Deputy Mayor's Office on Climate Change and Health; organizations such as Cidade Ativa in São Paulo, Brazil, looking to start up this work; health departments in London, U.K., and elsewhere interested in organizing Fit City conferences and mobilizing for change. The interest was wonderful, and a ringing endorsement for the types of interventions my colleagues and I were trying to make—but I was exhausted!

At first, I tried to consult at night and on weekends (which was possible thanks to the time difference between New York and places farther east), and during my four weeks of vacation time. Soon, though, I was completely worn out, and I knew the situation could not continue. And so, in 2013, I formally transitioned to the role of a part-time consultant. I told the City of New York I would still work for them but only part time, in the role of Senior Adviser for Active Living and Healthy Housing, which was the new name for the Built Environment and Active Design Program after Mayor Bill De Blasio's election. My consulting was challenging work, but so rewarding. It allowed me to see, firsthand, how others were taking the initiatives we'd tried so hard to implement in New York and applying them to their own challenges.

An Early Taste

Part of my excitement about transitioning to my new role no doubt stemmed from the fact that I already knew what it was going to involve. During my tenure in New York, I'd often been called upon to help other cities adopt and adapt our initiatives around health and the built environment for their own purposes.

In May 2011, for example, I'd traveled to New Orleans for the national convention of the American Institute of Architects (AIA). But I was doing double duty: the New York chapter of the AIA, along with staff from the Department of Health and Mental Hygiene, was hosting a Fit Nation conference annexed to the convention. This would be the second of the Fit Nation conferences my team was organizing as part of the peer-to-peer mentoring program on improving our built environments to address obesity that we had received funding from the U.S. CDC to do. Involved in this CDC grant initiative were fourteen local health departments located across the U.S.—west coast, east coast, midwest, the south; small, large, urban, suburban, even rural and tribal communities—that had signed up for mentoring on the built environment and health by the New York City Department of Health and Mental Hygiene. The gathering in New Orleans would bring three different professional sector partners from each of these cities together.

I had been to New Orleans only once before, for an American Planning Association national conference held there just as the city was beginning to rebuild after the devastation of Hurricane Katrina. This time, I would be there with my team—including Wendy Feuer, Skye Duncan, and Joyce Lee—and with the leaders and staff of three different departments from each of the fourteen mentee U.S. cities and counties, all attending the conference we'd spent months organizing.

Kate Rube had been hired using mentoring grant dollars that flowed from the CDC to the New York City Health Department's Built Environment and Active Design Program for advancing Active Design strategies, interventions, and evaluations across the country. Kate was organized, hardworking, always professional, and collaborative. She'd sorted out the logistics and booked the group of approximately fifty people, including our guest speakers, into the Marriott Hotel at the edge of the French Quarter, and had also booked a conference room at the convention hotel. She'd worked with New York's AIA chapter to alert other AIA chapters across the country about our one-day conference.

On the day after our arrival, Wendy, Skye, and I had an early-morning webinar. A few weeks prior, I had received an invitation from the World Health Organization's Pan American Health Organization (PAHO) office. Could I bring the intersectoral New York City team responsible for the Active Design Guidelines to Bogotá, Colombia, to help with training they were conducting for Ministry of Health staff from multiple Latin American countries on addressing non-communicable diseases? Unfortunately, the dates overlapped with our New Orleans conference. Undeterred, they'd asked about the possibility of a webinar. So there we were, presenting the health overview and evidence, then the planning and community-scale interventions and policies to consider implementing, and then the transportation and street-scale interventions and policies to consider implementing. The web technology employed by PAHO glitched from the very start, and we resorted to using the phone to present. We ended by answering questions from the audience, and we all took turns piping up to answer questions initially directed to one presenter or another.

When the webinar was over, Wendy, Skye, and I walked over to the conference room next door. Kate was already standing at the front of the large room with the agenda for the morning projected on the screen behind her. She had asked everyone to introduce themselves, identify which city or county they were from, and share what they did in their organizations. Over the course of the day, we would meet staff from the health departments of each city or county and their counterparts in transportation, planning, parks, and/or the advocacy and community groups the health departments had invited to join them.

When Kate and I had first met to start planning this conference, we had gone over our budget for travel costs. I had told Kate that I wanted three, or at the very least two, departments or stakeholder groups represented from each city or county. We would not provide funding for more than one health department staff member. We would not provide funding for more than one staff member from any one department in each city or county. The collaboration and partnerships among different departments and stakeholders had been key to our success in New York City, and I was convinced the same would be true in the cities we were now mentoring. It was clear among those cities that had already made good progress in their work that these partnerships had been critical. As a result, we now sat in a room with representation from three departments in each city or county. We would learn later that, despite working in the same place, some of them had met each other for the first time at the group dinner in New Orleans the night before.

Kate had arranged for guest speakers to come to our workshop, to present on topics in which the cities being mentored had expressed an interest. Kate and I picked the speakers for topics that overlapped based on top picks from the largest numbers of our participants. Many who were being mentored, for example, were interested in how to communicate with members of the public about the links of the built environment to health. Thus, one of our speakers spoke about media representations on the topic and how to better reach public audiences to build awareness and political support.

Next up was working exercises. We organized two different working sessions in which breakout groups would be charged with problem-solving around built environment and health policy and practice issues relevant to their communities. Again, we picked our topics from survey responses about what our participants were working on, or interested in working on. One breakout group had the people from each city working together with those from neighboring cities on problem-solving exercises. Another had those of similar professions from different cities working together. The idea was to start to create a network of professionals from the same sector—transportation, parks, planning—who would leave the conference with peers they could call as they worked on addressing health from a built environment perspective within their own sectors. For those communities where the different sectors had never worked together—or even met prior to this conference—the exercises were also designed to get them problem-solving together. Challenges could be shared; problems could be jointly solved with peers within and outside each participant's own city or county.

When we evaluated our participants later, we learned that many of them had been initially wary of joining our peer-mentoring network. Now comfortable enough to voice their opinions, many respondents told us they had been concerned that time would be wasted on pointless meetings and conference calls. But, as we would hear over and over later on, the calls, the Fit Nation conferences (an expanded Fit City encompassing not the stakeholders of one city but of multiple cities coming together to share their challenges, lessons, and opportunities), the webinars, and the connection with peers doing the same work (who were willing to share their successes and failures) were incredibly useful. When the CDC visited New York to hear about the peer-mentoring work they were funding, we heard a very validating comment from one of the officers: "This was the best money CDC ever spent."

Unfortunately, once the federal stimulus funds had been spent and the two-year grant ended, the continuation of the peer-mentoring network—though strongly requested by all fourteen cities working with our program, as well as additional communities that heard about us later—was terminated. The CDC no longer provided funds. Attempts by me and others to engage foundation funders to continue and expand this important work was also met with silence, or with comments such as "We don't fund what has already been tried." But what if what has been tried actually works? It's a question, and an issue, that needs further attention if this work is to continue and to grow.

As frustrating as the long-term outcome of the peer-mentoring program was to all concerned, the experience gave me an encouraging taste of what it would be like to work in a consulting role. I loved the idea of sharing what I knew with others, and of helping them to do what they could to get similar programs off the ground. Which is why I was happy to travel to Canada in October 2012 to offer another assist.

———

Skye Duncan, Wendy Feuer, and I—among others—are being shepherded through different neighborhoods in the Region of Peel. Located to the west and northwest of Toronto, Ontario, the region's approximately 463 square miles is home to some 1.4 million people and to a great number of businesses large and small. Although often thought of as part of the suburbs of Toronto, the Peel Region has three municipalities: Mississauga, Brampton, and Caledon. Part of the region, like Mississauga, actually has its own downtown core, and a host of business, education, and housing opportunities for its residents. Other areas, like Caledon, are much more residential and rural. In 2012 I had been hired part time by the region as a consultant, and had in turn mobilized some of my New York City colleagues to participate in this endeavor to help Peel Region to become a fitter place. I had also brought in Andy Stone from the Trust for Public Land for his expertise in children's play spaces, and Candace Young (who earlier worked with Sabrina Baronberg on New York City's healthy bodega initiative), now at Philadelphia's Food Trust, for her expertise in food initiatives.

We were on a mission to assist Peel to improve its environments for physical activity and healthier food access amid the growth and development occurring in its three municipalities. Rapid suburban growth in the population of this region on the outskirts of Toronto was presenting both opportunities and challenges for addressing the health of the region's residents. Although Peel Public Health had at first asked me to deliver the keynote address at their Healthy Peel by Design conference individually, I had, during the planning process, suggested a cross-sector panel, one meant to explicitly illustrate the important role of the other government sectors and players in this work. Thus, I had suggested a panel that included Wendy and Skye, among others, following the opening speech by their Medical Officer of Health, Dr. David Mowat, whom I'd known since my Public Health and Preventive Medicine residency training years in Toronto. The animated discussions among those of us on the panel would prove success-ful in exciting not only the public health staff present but also the staff and leadership of the other Peel regional and municipal government departments that had been invited.

We'd spent the day prior to the conference on a bus, touring the region. We passed through and into residential developments by way of multi-lane roads that accommodated the fast-moving automobiles all around us but left no room for bicycles or transit. We would hear about the paucity of public transport options. We would see sidewalks present, but either vast distances or unpleas-ant, boring surroundings for the pedestrian. Not surprisingly, few pedestrians were seen. We would drive past strip malls and big-box stores with large parking lots separating the entryways from the sidewalks. Many of these parking lots had ample empty spots. Some of the strip malls and stores had residential developments within a walkable distance, but given the layout of the roads and the developments, it was not surprising that we saw few if any people walking to the stores.

In the course of the bus ride that day, and during the conference lunch and dinner events, we would meet Janet Menard, commis-sioner of Human Services, and her staff. Janet—tall, blond, dressed in perfectly tailored power suits—would tell us that her staff was about to embark on updating the guidelines for affordable hous-ing in Peel Region. I told her about our recently completed study—*Active Design: Affordable Designs for Affordable Housing*—that showed just how affordable and feasible it was to integrate many Active Design strategies into affordable housing. This would be an oppor-tunity, she said, to make affordable housing routinely healthier in our municipalities. The commissioner of Health Services, Janette Smith, and Peel Public Health agreed to be partners on the project. True to its word and intentions, and with the help of a few New Yorkers like myself, Peel Region released its Affordable Housing Active Design Guidelines and Standards in 2014.

First Up: Miami

Miami, it turns out, is hot even in January. I fussed with my black blazer and black skirt, wishing I were more suitably attired for the weather—perhaps in shorts and a tank top . . . on the beach! But it was only a passing thought. Unrequited dreams of sand and surf aside, I was happy to be just where I was, preparing to deliver the keynote address at the first of what would become an annual Fit City Miami conference. It was early in 2013, and I had spent the last half of 2012 helping Cheryl Jacobs from the Miami chapter of the American Institute of Architects and Karen Hamilton from the county's planning department get the conference off the ground. I had been connected to them in a myriad of ways, not the least of which was the CDC mentoring grant. Miami-Dade County's Health Department had been one of New York City health department's built environment and health mentees.

The room we'd been given at the downtown campus of Miami-Dade College had high ceilings and a number of large, round conference tables facing the podium and stage. From my position behind the microphone, I could see that the space was nearly full, with more than a hundred health, architecture, planning, and environmental sustainability professionals and students. The previous year, in a test run for this gathering, I had spoken to a much smaller crowd in a much smaller room, but the topic had been the same: how to work across sectors to create more options for healthy choices for Miami area residents. That gathering had gone well, and the main event was now upon us.

Our Fit City conferences in New York had evolved to include site tours and field visits—from the activity-promoting pathways of High Line Park, to the stairs at the Cooper Union Academic Building that grace the front cover of the *Active Design Guidelines*, to Arbor House. Cheryl and Karen had decided that they wanted to offer a tour of one site in Miami.

Leading our group on the walkabout was Bernard Zyscovich,

principal and founder of Zyscovich Architects. I'd met Bernard,
both architect and urban planner, several years earlier, when his
firm became a sponsor of a South Florida U.S Green Building
Council event. I was there to introduce green building professionals and architects in the area to the need and opportunities
for working together to concurrently address the health of our
environment and the health of our children and adults through
building infrastructure and developments. I had talked about
the LEED Innovation Credit for Physical Activity that we were
developing at that time. Bernard introduced himself and we'd
stayed in touch, bound by our common professional interests.

Those interested in the tour joined Bernard at a new building
a short walk from our main conference venue. At the time, the
Wolfson Building was not yet open to the public, but it was very
nearly complete. Bernard's firm had designed this building using
the LEED Innovation Credit for Physical Activity, and they were
rightly proud of their work. A grand open staircase greeted us as
we entered. We would ascend and descend many stairs during
that tour, not only the grand staircase but the many other fire
stairs that were flooded with sunlight and would be easily accessible for student and faculty use. I would sometimes join Bernard
at the front of the tour; other times, I would fall back to watch
the crowds. And I would find myself thinking how far we had
come. It seemed not so long ago that the LEED Innovation Credit
for Physical Activity didn't even exist. It was not so long ago at all
that Active Design itself was an unknown concept. And here I
was, touring one of the over 250 buildings that were now using
the LEED credit that I had played a part in creating.

Road Trip: Singapore, Malaysia, and Canada

February 2013. It had taken months of planning, but I was finally
departing on a one-month trip that would take me to four
Australian cities, then to Singapore and Malaysia, and finally to

Winnipeg, Manitoba. It was Friday, February 1. The first leg of the journey was New York to Los Angeles, followed by a connecting flight that would get me to Melbourne—a total of twenty-one hours of flying time, nearly thirty if you added in the time spent waiting at airports.

I landed in Melbourne in the middle of the afternoon on Sunday, February 3. Dr. Billie Giles-Corti—whose name I'd heard many times during my disease detective days when research on the built environment and health from Down Under was cited—would be at the airport to pick me up. I'd met Billie in my early years in New York City. She'd been on sabbatical then, touring U.S. cities to learn about the work being done to translate built-environment and physical-activity evidence into policies and practices. We'd had lunch and discussed Billie's research and my work in translating research such as hers into policy and practice. A few years later, we met up in New York again, this time with Billie's colleague Dr. Carolyn Whitzman, an urban planning professor originally from Toronto and now working at the University of Melbourne. Carolyn, Billie, and I had dreamed up a workshop on health and urban planning that would address physical activity as well as safety, particularly for women, around the world. Carolyn, who had previously been a consultant to the United Nations, submitted our ideas to the UN, and we ended up with an invitation to present the workshop at the World Urban Forum in Naples, Italy, in 2012.

Now, I could see Billie waving as I exited the arrivals area of Melbourne airport. She gave me a little hug, and then reached over to take my suitcase. I followed as she pulled it along, leading me out into the heat—it was summer in the southern hemisphere. We crossed the pedway to the parkade and embarked on a little tour of Melbourne. Billie brought me down to an area by the Yarra River that had in recent years been redeveloped to include a large pedestrian plaza. People would sit and sun themselves there during the day; movies were sometimes shown at sundown; musicians often played. A little farther along the river were food stalls, and we decided to grab a bite. I had not slept for about twenty-four hours and was a little dazed, but Billie was adamant that it was best to stay awake and acclimatize to my new time zone. I stuck it out, and eventually we made our way to meet several others for dinner, including those from the Heart Foundation who had joined forces across their chapters to bring me here.

The next few days would find me presenting my New York and U.S. work to a wide variety of audiences—public health officials, a mixed audience with planners and architects, and city planning and city hall staff. I tried to tailor my message for the different stakeholders. For public health, my main task was to talk about how to do this work, how to engage sectors outside of health and get their buy-in. For the mixed audience with planners and architects, I needed to convince them that they played a critical role in the creation of buildings, streets, and neighborhoods that would help enable people who wanted to make healthy choices to do so—affordably, and with less difficulty than they might imagine. With the city planning and city hall staff, I talked about the opportunities to integrate health into the greening priorities of the city, and stressed the value of doing so.

The response was overwhelmingly positive. People listened intently and asked well-considered questions. You could tell they were serious about learning whatever I had come to share. You could tell there was a strong likelihood that the ideas from New York would be taken up here, too. It was exciting to see how far the work had come in a mere seven years.

From Melbourne, I flew to Sydney, where I was met by Peter McCue. In many ways, Peter was my Australian counterpart. One of my main jobs in New York had been to corral the leaders of different city departments, private sector architects and developers, and community advocates to improve our environments for health, particularly as they related to the obesity and non-communicable disease epidemics. Peter had a similar job in Sydney, in the state of New South Wales. He was the executive director of the Premier's Council for Active Living. In June 2012, Peter had attended the Fit City 7 Conference. Soon after, he'd reached out with an invitation to assist the Australian cities with their goal of improving opportunities and choices for active living. A new governor had just been elected in New South Wales, and though Peter himself had not yet had a chance to meet with him, he ensured that I did. He was eager to fill the new administration in on what was being done in the rest of the world, and to encourage policy-makers to not let New South Wales fall behind.

Peter had also enlisted my help to organize the first of what would become an annual Fit New South Wales Conference, which was debuting during my visit. On a bright sunny morning, the air crisp and refreshing, Peter picked me up from my hotel and shuttled me to the government hall. I helped him open the conference by sharing my work and experiences on Fit City conferences, and on initiatives that created more options for physical activity and for active transportation in New York, in other U.S. cities, and elsewhere. I then sat on a panel with Australian presenters, among them a developer of new suburbs in the Sydney metropolitan area who was working with Peter's team to change what this type of development looked like. These suburbs would have not only sidewalks but walking trails; they would be located along existing or planned transit stops; and they would include shops that people could walk to, lessening the dependency on cars. The developer added that the new development was so far selling out faster than any of the previous suburbs he had helped create.

With our work in Sydney done, Peter decided he would accompany me on the next leg of my trip. We were off to Canberra, Australia's capital, where we would be hosted by the

Australian National Public Health Agency (ANPHA). At the ANPHA office the next morning, I presented to and then sat down in problem-solving meetings with their researchers, national staff, and local Canberra health department leadership. There I would meet Dr. Paul Kelly, chief health officer for Canberra. Paul would later come to New York on sabbatical to study our policies for obesity and to make comparisons with Canberra's work in this field. I would send him references and information for his report on New York. We would end up writing a paper together.

Next up: Perth. I arrived on a Friday, checked in to my hotel, and had a good night's sleep. The next morning, the Australian Heart Foundation's Trevor Shelton picked me up and showed me around the city, including areas that were already under development and others slated for new development. We saw newly created bicycle lanes. We saw train stations where the tracks had been put underground to facilitate additional ground-level space for shopping, retail, and housing. We went to the nearby seaside town of Fremantle for a lunch of fresh fish, followed by a walk along its historic streets.

The next day, a Sunday, Billie, who happened to be back in her hometown for a visit, picked me up and drove me out to the beach with her Sunday morning swimming group. I was a little daunted, hearing Billie tell the story of record high numbers of great white shark attacks the previous year in Perth waters—about one attack per month, instead of the usual one per year. Nobody knew the reason for the change, though theories abounded about low fish stocks, warmer waters, and other possible factors. I wondered whether I should just sit on the beach and watch the others swim, but once we arrived, I couldn't resist the clear, warm, blue-green waters. One of Billie's swimming friends was Dr. Fiona Bull, university professor and incoming president of the International Society of Physical Activity and Public Health. Fiona would later invite me to present on the built environment to the health round-table at her biennial international conference in São Paulo.

Australia had been an absolute whirlwind: meeting after meeting, coffees and lunches and dinners with like-minded people, contacts made and partnerships formed. On my next flight—from Perth to Kuala Lumpur—my brain was practically buzzing! I was so excited by the opportunities cropping up all around me, and by the enthusiasm for this work that was so important to our health and well-being. My consulting career was off to a rip-roaring start, and I was only partway through my first big trip.

After a late first night of dining on rotis and curry with my cousin Nick and his family, I got right to work scouting potential projects for a World Health Organization (WHO) publication. Prior to my arrival, I'd reached out to a company called Sime Darby, referred by one of my contacts in Perth. I was hopeful that perhaps Sime Darby, a major developer in Malaysia, could provide a case study for the WHO publication. And so, I met with one of the company's vice-presidents, who graciously drove me to see several of their developments. She was clearly (and rightly!) proud of these projects, which intentionally included parks and playgrounds, walking paths, and bicycle lanes, with the aim of both greening the environment and offering healthy recreation opportunities for residents. But when we finished our tour, we found ourselves stuck in traffic on the one main highway that connected several of these developments to the city center. And it wasn't as if we'd had a choice about our mode of travel: there was no other way to get to the main city—no public transit, no bike paths, nothing. The challenge, I noted, was that these suburban developments would only promote active recreation opportunities. Active transportation wasn't an option here.

My final stop before returning to North America was Singapore. When Wendy Feuer and Skye Duncan had learned that I was visiting relatives in Singapore, they'd put me in touch with their architectural and planning colleagues there. Could I do a presentation for them on the work of the New York City Active Design Guidelines team? After all, the guidelines had been named as a reason—along with a variety of initiatives in planning and transportation—for the Singaporean government awarding New York City the World City Prize in 2012. Singapore had inaugurated the prestigious prize in 2010 in an effort to identify and recognize cities that, though at one point in decline, managed to use smart government policies, good planning, and architecture to recover and even revitalize themselves. The first award had gone to Bilbao, Spain.

In addition to my presentation to the group, I took part in meetings with the leadership and staff of Singapore's Ministry of Health, meetings that helped pave the way for the intersectoral development of a Master Plan for Healthy Living in Singapore. And the WHO Centre for Health Development in Kobe, Japan— for which urban health issues is a main focus—had contacted me in January to see if I'd be able to find a case study for healthy urban planning in Asia. Their request was still fresh in my mind, and I requested a tour of developments that the built environment professionals and government would consider prime examples.

The morning after my presentation, meetings, and media interviews, I was on my way with my colleagues from the Ministry of Health to meet their counterparts in the housing ministry. In Singapore, the vast majority—over 80 percent—of residents live in housing made affordable by some type of government program. Every development we visited had playgrounds for children and outdoor exercise equipment. Every development had nearby shops, cafés, and transit stations or stops. Some had community vegetable gardens and solar panels, and some captured rainwater on their roofs. It was so exciting to see smart growth and transit-oriented development at play, routinely integrated into every development I was seeing.

If you were looking for a way to send a body into shock, boarding a plane in a Singaporean summer and deboarding into a Canadian winter would be pretty high on the list. Smack in the middle of the Canadian Prairies, Winnipeg, Manitoba, is a city of about 700,000 residents. Head a bit farther north and you reach small towns like Churchill, known in part for its polar bear–watching adventures. Needless to say, winters in these parts are very cold.

Weather aside, I was happy to be there. The Manitoba chapter of the Canadian Institute of Planners (CIP) had invited me to their annual conference to run a public engagement workshop on healthy development, and I had been helping them to plan it for the last several months, via conference calls. I'd encouraged them to reach out to the health department in their Regional Health Authority, in particular to those there who were involved in the Heart and Stroke Foundation's Healthy Canada by Design initiative. All of that intersectoral planning was about to pay off. In April 2013, Winnipeg Regional Health Authority staff members Sarah Prowse and Deanna Betteridge would write about how they'd met and developed relationships with planners and other City of Winnipeg staff, and learned about current City projects that presented opportunities to promote active living. A dialogue had been created, they said, around ways in which the health authority could be involved in this work. "We have now been formally invited to sit at the *OurWinnipeg* implementation table for the City's Complete Community Strategy," they concluded, noting that it was a huge step for an external organization since they worked for the Regional Health Authority and not the city of Winnipeg, per se. "All of these developments have been unexpected outcomes that have grown out of our

involvement in the Active Design workshop. While the initial outcome was the delivery of a workshop, the relationships developed
through the process have laid the foundation for our work with
the City of Winnipeg." A few years on, the City of Winnipeg
webpage prominently features two key initiatives: public engagement, and pedestrian and cycling strategies. Even today, Walk
Bike Projects feature on their homepage. Sarah and Deanna
may not have expected the outcomes we achieved through the
workshop, but I had. Having done this type of partnership work
in other cities, I was certainly hopeful that it could occur in
Winnipeg, too. Perhaps Sarah and Deanna hadn't heard me
when I mentioned these outcomes during our planning sessions.
Or perhaps they hadn't quite believed me, until they saw it happen in their own city.

An Olympic-Sized Effort

I am looking forward to my meeting with Dr. Lesley Mountford,
director of Public Health for London's North East Side and the
Borough of Hackney. Lesley and I have had more conference
calls than I can count as I've helped her to organize the inaugural Fit City London conference, but this will be our first face-to-
face since I met her at New York's Fit City 7 conference in 2012.

It's March 2013 and I'm enjoying a rare sunny-day walk along
the Thames River, on my way to meet Lesley for lunch. I'm curious to hear about one of her last-minute plans for the event, and
about the city's adoption of New York's "Burn Calories, Not
Electricity. Take the Stairs!" signs. But I'm especially looking
forward to the tour Lesley has arranged of the facilities built
for the 2012 Summer Olympics. Lesley and I had talked often
over the last few years about the challenges of being an Olympic
host city, and she'd shared how hard her City of London design
and building colleagues were working to avoid the most common pitfall experienced by a myriad of other cities after hosting

Olympic and Pan-American Games: million- to billion-dollar infrastructures left unused or underused once the Games left town.

It's no secret that the Olympic Games are expensive. An Associated Press analysis pegged the cost of the 2018 Winter Games in Pyeongchang, South Korea, at $12.9 billion, and the 2016 Summer Games in Rio de Janeiro at $13.1 billion. A huge part of those costs goes toward the construction of infrastructure—state-of-the-art stadiums and facilities, athletes' villages, and the transportation systems needed to shuttle spectators to and from events. All too often, that spending goes to waste; a Brazilian attendee at Fit City 7 in New York spoke of the distant, isolated stadium built for the 1963 Pan American Games in São Paulo, now fallen into disrepair, its grounds overgrown with long grasses and weeds.

Done right, however, all of that spending can be an investment for the post-Olympic future. In 2008, Beijing wisely built three new subway lines to facilitate transportation during the Games—lines that are now used by the city's residents, easing both traffic congestion and the resulting smog, and promoting the extra physical activity that comes from walking to and from the transit stops.

London wanted to do it right, and planning for its Olympic legacy was on the agenda from the very start. Now, as part of the Fit City conference, London wanted to show us what it had achieved. Lesley and I also wanted to use the recent games to highlight the importance of physical activity—and of physical infrastructure that creates opportunities and options for activity for all.

And so, on day two of the conference, a large group of us—foreign and local—accompany Lesley's staff on a walking tour of the developments constructed for the 2012 Summer Olympic Games. We can see the stadiums and sports facilities dotting the skyline, but that's not our focus. Instead, we check out the athletes' housing that's scheduled to be converted into a variety of mixed-income and affordable housing apartment complexes, so nicely near to those state-of-the-art recreational facilities. We see the surrounding grounds with walking trails and parks where outdoor play areas—from ping-pong tables made of concrete to children's playgrounds—have been added. We see new walking trails that have sprung up over what were once open sewers. What's especially interesting to note is that all of these improvements are smack in the middle of the previously impoverished district of London's East End. The city had made a conscious choice to build its Olympic stadium and facilities there, and to use this construction to also create new parks, new housing, and new transportation connections to the rest of the city. It's a model of how things can be, with forethought and planning, and I smile as I see my fellow conference participants—some of whom have joined us from cities about to host their own events—taking notes. This is the best possible way to spread the word.

The question now is where we go from here. With all of this support, how can we ensure that we'll finally see the lasting change we so desperately need?

CONCLUSION

WHAT'S NEXT?

Life can only be understood backwards; but it must be lived forwards.

—KIERKEGAARD

The best way to predict the future is to create it.

—ABRAHAM LINCOLN

IN A DISASTER, people walk. They walk because they have to. Cars are often ordered off the roads and public transportation often has to shut down, even if temporarily.

Extreme weather events are occurring more and more frequently. The threat of terrorist attacks, and terrorist attacks themselves, in the Western world have also been on the rise. Many of us remember seeing on television the long lines of yellow school buses and cars and campers trying to get out of the most heavily affected areas in New Orleans during Hurricane Katrina. More recently, during Hurricane Sandy in New York City, power outages in the most ravaged areas of the city, such as the Rockaways, had residents of old-style social housing towers trapped on high floors because they were unable or too afraid to use the completely dark stairwells without any natural light. Many New York City government employees volunteered to walk, run, or rollerblade to find those whose homes had been destroyed by the storm, or who had no electricity in their buildings, so they could provide assistance.

In a recent severe snowstorm in January 2016, with record-breaking snowfalls, New York State Governor Andrew Cuomo mandated that cars remain off the roads. Public transportation rail tracks iced over and those lines had to be shut down. My neighbors and I, however, were not stuck without food or water. Although many of us had purchased non-perishable foods and filled up our bathtubs and pots and water jugs, or loaded up on bottled water, our neighborhood was spared from any power outage or water shutoff. Television news stories showed neighborhood stores whose owners and staff lived nearby and were able to open up for people living within walking distance, and that was the case with our nearby supermarket. Children and their parents who lived within walking distance of parks, especially parks with hills, ended up enjoying the snowy days with sledding and tobogganing. In contrast, those who had no amenities within walkable distances were trapped on their properties, hoping the storm would abate before any food they had stockpiled ran out.

I had not yet moved to New York City in 2001, but we all know stories about what happened on the morning of 9/11 when the Twin Towers fell. One woman I know worked on a high floor of a high-rise building in midtown Manhattan near the Empire State Building. She told me how she and her office colleagues watched on a small TV screen in the office as the first tower fell, and then the second, bringing the realization that this was no accident. A terrorist attack was happening right in their midst, just south of where they were. People ran down the stairs of the building and out onto the streets. They tried their cellphones to call their loved ones but the phone lines were overloaded, with so many others trying to do the same. People feared what could happen if they went into the subway. Many decided they would walk home. They hoped their loved ones would and could do the same.

Disasters, both natural and human-made, illustrate for us just how important it is that our homes, schools, workplaces, and grocery stores be at walkable distances from each other. This allows us to stay alive, healthy, fit, and with our loved ones when our cars and our public transportation systems cannot be relied upon. Which inevitably happens, sooner or later.

The work to create healthy built environments continues, and its successes are outstanding, in New York City and around the world. This is excellent news when we consider what it portends for the aftermath of disasters, and for the more insidious destruction caused to millions of lives yearly from obesity, physical inactivity, and unhealthy diets.

One of the key successes of the Active Design movement has been the growth of active transportation initiatives. Even before this book was released, my friend Sam Schwartz published *Street Smart: The Rise of Cities and the Fall of Cars.* A former commissioner in the New York City Department of Transportation and a transportation engineer by training, Sam spent a couple of hours with me one afternoon in his sunny boardroom in downtown Manhattan discussing the most important health issues today, and what his transportation engineering firm, Sam Schwartz Engineering, is doing, with a special focus on walkability, to make a difference. It is truly remarkable that a growing number of urban planning, design, and transportation engineering firms all over the world—from the forerunner, Jan Gehl of Copenhagen, to other international giants like AECOM and Stantec—are making active transportation a key part of their work. Well, one might say, with all the problems plaguing our cities today—from global warming to terrorism threats to obesity and non-communicable disease epidemics to the need for the economic revitalization of blighted urban districts to the needs of an aging population in many of our towns and cities—how could they not?

I now also regularly attend full-house public events where active transportation is the main subject. What started as a focus just for professionals and a few members of the public at our Fit City conferences has now become a topic that energizes many who work in the transportation and planning worlds, and inspires an increasing number of public events and book readings.

On March 9, 2016, I was at just such an event. Janette Sadik-Khan, former New York City Transportation commissioner, was going to be discussing her work on creating an "urban revolution" on and through city streets. To get to the event, I walked past many of the lasting infrastructure interventions the New York City Department of Transportation (DOT) had instituted during Janette's time: striped crossings on narrowed streets, additional pedestrian spaces created with paint and plant potters, bicycle lanes painted in green, a large bicycle-share station with its bright-blue Citi Bikes. I arrived early, and good thing, too. There were probably a couple of hundred seats at the Barnes and Noble in Union Square, and I just managed to nab one before it was too late. Part of the reason for the excited crowd was that Janette was going to be on stage in conversation with David Byrne, the iconic singer, bike advocate . . . and designer of some city bicycle racks that were cool and quintessentially New York, like the one shaped like a red high-heeled shoe in front of the Bergdorf Goodman department store.

That night, Janette said many of the things that I have said in this book. She described her work as a daily fight to give people more choices, and pointed out that New York City created a model that any city can follow.

Successes in fighting the obesity epidemic are already being achieved by cities that have spent the last decade (or even less) in policy and practice efforts to improve their physical and food environments, so that more options and choices are made available to their residents and visitors for physical activity and healthy eating. After more than three decades of unrelenting rise, childhood obesity trends are now reversing in U.S. cities like New York, Philadelphia, and San Diego. After a mere decade of concerted efforts by public health professionals working in partnership with other government departments, professionals from other sectors, non-government organizations, community advocates, and individuals with the power to change the daily environments in which we work, go to school, play, and perhaps pray, we are starting to beat this modern-day public health epidemic. In New York City, physical inactivity in adults has also gone down in recent years, after a decade of no significant change. Adult obesity in New York State has also shown a recent reversal.

The successes that are being achieved in transforming our physical environment, however, are shadowed by insufficient progress on these issues in the developing world, particularly and most crucially in the increasingly developed and urban areas that are aspiring to become great cities in Latin America, Africa, China, India, and other Asian countries. Unfortunately, all too often these rapidly growing cities are modeling themselves on an outdated idea of Western cities; by replicating the car-dependent model, they find themselves increasingly plagued by traffic congestion and traffic-related deaths, air pollution, obesity, and noncommunicable diseases. Active transportation policies and practices still need a great deal of work in these regions.

Additionally, although many cities in the developed world have begun to address active and sustainable transportation choices, the car is still the predominant mode of transportation, particularly in many cities in North America and Australia. And many cities still need to do much more on the issue of supporting choices for activity in buildings, and using government policy to address healthy food access and unhealthy food exposure. Although health departments across North America are increasingly working with corner store owners and operators to increase healthy options, too few cities are working on policies to improve zoning and tax incentives in order to ensure meaningful access to supermarkets, farmers' markets, and community gardens in food desert neighborhoods. More cities need to follow the lead of Detroit, with its policy banning fast food restaurants around schools, and use city zoning policies to decrease our children's unhealthy food exposure when parents are not around to help them make good choices. Like New York, other cities can also look at what policies governing food, physical activity, and screen time in daycares can be developed, implemented, and enforced. These settings-based building-scale and food issues have generally received less attention currently in the design and planning of cities than active transportation issues.

Though the progress has been encouraging, we still have a long way to go to bring obesity rates in both children and adults back to pre-1960s levels. Fortunately, since the release of the Active Design Guidelines, a whole set of second-phase—and even third-phase—initiatives in the movement for physical environmental change are afoot.

I first met Yianice Hernandez when she was director of research for Green Communities at Enterprise Community Partners, a non-profit organization started by an American developer and his wife, Jim and Patty Rouse, in 1982. The vision of the organization is to give everyone a decent, affordable home, and its key goal is to improve the quality of affordable housing in the United States, integrating environmentally sustainable "green" features into new developments. Shampa Chanda and Bea De la Torre, assistant commissioners in the New York City Department of Housing Preservation and Development (HPD) and key contacts for the work related to the Active Design Guidelines and their implementation, had recommended to me that I meet with Enterprise: "We already require all HPD-funded affordable housing projects to use Enterprise Green Communities criteria, so you should see how you can get them to integrate more health and Active Design criteria."

One factor for success in cross-sector collaboration is listening to advice. I never tell my colleagues, who are experts in their own sectors, what I think they have to do. What I can do, however, is share with them what I know of the data and evidence concerning public health issues, including what has worked elsewhere and what studies have shown will lead to improvement in health outcomes. I also share whatever I discover that might be of benefit to their work. Strategies that can improve maintenance and decrease maintenance costs of the buildings and housing developments? Check. Strategies that can improve affordable housing residents' access to necessary items like food, and especially healthy food? Check. I may even help them with creating public engagement initiatives, using health as a shared value among the public to lead the conversations for environmental change. Then, I wait. I may prod with emails and with questions at every meeting about what we could possibly and feasibly do within their departments and fields. But I always wait for their answers. And so, when I'm asked by other jurisdictions whether I faced opposition from other sectors to my work in New York, I am able to answer, definitively, "No." You don't tend to see opposition from others to the ideas that are their own.

The other critical factor for success is this: once I get advice, I always follow up.

I asked HPD for introductions to their Enterprise Green Communities contacts and searched for information on their website. Now my staff and I were on the lookout for people from that organization when we attended meetings on housing issues, and we sent emails to housing developers who might have contacts there. And we found Yianice Hernandez.

Now, I had to get Enterprise Green Communities on board.

Yianice and I met in her office in Manhattan, a bright, airy space with simple, contemporary furnishings that reminded me of the U.S. Green Building Council (USGBC) headquarters in Washington, D.C. With long, dark hair down to her mid-back and Woody Allen–style glasses, Yianice looked like a cross between a trendy singer and an academic. She explained that Enterprise Green Communities was an organization working to unconventionally integrate environmental issues into the social cause of housing those in need, with typically very limited budgets. And yes, they were indeed in the process of updating their Enterprise Green Communities Criteria and would welcome more health-related criteria for supporting and promoting the health and well-being of affordable housing residents.

Another key strategy for partnering successfully is sharing the workload. The last thing a potential partner wants to hear is that your request will turn into a burden for their already over-busy staff and organization. But if your requests for help come with an offer of staffing resources and extra capacity? That is a much better prospect. Yianice was delighted to hear that I could also offer her practical staff support. We had recently engaged Angela Aloia, a Presidential Fellow for the U.S. Department of Housing and Urban Development, to work with our team, and Angela could engage in the necessary but painstaking work of integrating the Active Design Guidelines strategies into the appropriate sections of the Enterprise Green Communities criteria for new construction of affordable housing. I am happy to report that our partnership was very successful and the new, merged criteria were released.

Incentives for Certification

It's May 2015. I am in Washington, D.C., and it is a beautiful sunny Saturday. I have arrived a day and a half early, taking advantage of a ride-sharing opportunity, for the WELL Building Standard Advisory Meeting that will be taking place on May 11 and 12 at the USGBC headquarters. This meeting will be another second-phase initiative following on the growing awareness of and interest in health among architects and building professionals who were exposed to these ideas through the Active Design Guidelines, the LEED Innovation Credit for Physical Activity, and other first-phase initiatives.

The WELL Building Standard is a new building certification system for health and wellness created by the International WELL Building Institute, a public benefit company that has said it will reinvest over half of its profits in public benefit initiatives. It has made it its mission to improve health and well-being through the built environment, focusing first on the creation of healthier buildings. Like the Leadership in Energy and Environmental Design (LEED) green building certification system of the USGBC, WELL certification comes at a cost to the developer and building owner of tens of thousands of dollars. WELL is a market-driven tool, created by a former Wall Street banker who wanted to do some good using a business model. Although the USGBC is set up as a non-profit organization, while the International WELL Building Institute is a public benefits corporation, both use and rely on market principles. Companies pay a lot of money for certification, and that money in turn supports the certifying organizations' staff. While many residents of new affordable-housing buildings are chosen through a local government lottery process for the limited number of available spots, other clients are buying or renting units at market-value prices. The certifications buy bragging rights for building owners and developers when it comes to the environmental friendliness or healthiness of their buildings, which helps them attract higher-paying residents.

The WELL Building Standard meeting started early on a beautiful sunny day in Washington, and I was glad to have walked to the USGBC headquarters, close to the hotel where I was staying along with the other expert reviewers from across the United States. In a sunlit conference room, the dozen or so experts would be put to two days of intensive work with the WELL leadership and staff. WELL staff provided an overall orientation to the WELL Building Standard at morning sessions, and the experts all participated actively as we laboriously plowed through each section of the standard, focused on Indoor Air Quality, Mental Well-being, Fitness, and Nutrition, among others. Air quality experts and psychologists offered their input on the sections on indoor air quality and mental health factors and interventions. There were worksite-wellness providers present. There were design firms present. I was there to provide a lens on obesity and on its related chronic diseases, looking at physical activity and access to healthier foods and beverages. Joyce Lee, who had relocated to Philadelphia, was also present.

About two months after this meeting, I received an email from Sarah Welton. Sarah had approached me some time back when she was finishing up her master's degree to ask if I could spare some time to discuss career options with her. A fit triathlete, Sarah planned to work on healthier real estate developments, and after graduation she was hired by the WELL Building Institute. Sarah asked if I could assist WELL in a more intensive review of the section that she was charged with, Fitness, particularly by giving input into the research that would inform that section. I agreed, and reviewed for Sarah the research she had found, which she then used to create a document supporting the relevant criteria. Where there were gaps, I was able to help her add to her research data, and I put my experience to work, suggesting changes to the language in the hopes that reframing and rewording might increase the work's appeal and salience to its broad target audience.

It has been over three years since I completed that review, and now that WELL has decided to move into community-level factors and pilot a set of criteria for rating communities, my expertise might be helpful once again. And so I came to work again with WELL, this time with Sarah's colleague, Vienna McLeod, on the WELL Community Standard.

In order to be approved for construction in New York City, affordable housing developments with supports and funding from the Department of Housing Preservation and Development must now be Enterprise Green Communities certified. Although there are myriad mandatory and optional strategies to achieve certification, those mandatory strategies and a threshold of optional strategies must be integrated.

Outside of affordable housing, healthy building certification systems, while not mandatory, are gradually evolving. WELL now serves market-driven needs and desires in this realm, and a program called FitWel was previously initiated.

In 2012, while Joyce Lee was still at the City of New York, and while I was still the director of the New York City Department of Health and Mental Hygiene's Built Environment and Active Design Program, we both received an invitation to travel to Washington, D.C. After undertaking the myriad bureaucratic steps to get travel approvals from City administration, Joyce and I found ourselves sitting around a conference table with six or seven others in the windowless conference room of a large hotel. The meeting was being led by the U.S. General Services Administration (GSA). The U.S. Centers for Disease Control and Prevention (CDC) had also been invited. Joyce and I had been invited because of our work in New York in leading the development of the LEED Innovation Credit for Physical Activity (which had, in its latest iteration at the time, become the LEED pilot credit Design for Active Occupants, integrating physical activity and health strategies into the LEED green building rating system). We had also co-led with interested developers the development of a LEED Innovation Credit for Urban Agriculture, and I had worked on an Innovation Credit for Healthy Food and Beverage Access for our new health department headquarters.

We were told that the GSA wanted to do more to make federal government buildings and office facilities that it built and managed healthier for government staff. There was an opportunity to affect the lives of hundreds of thousands of federal government employees who spent at least some, if not most, of their time in these buildings and facilities. Leadership and staff of GSA had thought that perhaps a healthy-building certification system could be created to systematically track—and push—each building manager's implementation of health-promoting strategies. They wanted the CDC's help, and mine, to identify the evidence-based health strategies. And they wanted Joyce's and my experience in developing new healthy-building credits for LEED to inform their process. Since there was, at the start of the FitWel process, also a lack of building certification systems with a focus on health as the primary outcome, with WELL having not yet entered the market, our working group also envisioned that the FitWel process could begin with government buildings but eventually be extended to buildings outside the government sector. When I left the New York City health department in 2015, FitWel was in the process of being piloted in GSA, CDC, and City of New York government buildings. With the development of WELL as a market-driven tool released to the private sector, and with the 2015 Enterprise Green Communities criteria available for Affordable Housing and now intentionally integrating a comprehensive overlay of health criteria including Active Design criteria, the role of FitWel has become less clear. At the time of the writing of this book, WELL reported having 2,146 projects impacting 383 million square feet of real estate in 51 countries, while FitWel reported having 210 projects certified or pending certification.

Work to improve our physical environments for the prevention of obesity and non-communicable disease is taking place also, increasingly, on the international front. And it is much needed.

Working on the Built Environment Around the World

It is pouring rain, a heavy, tropical rain, and all of us in the van are wondering whether we can make a dash to the St. George University building for our workshop without getting soaked. Tall palm trees lining the driveway where we are parked sway in the warm, wet winds. We decide to wait it out, since we're a bit early, but I'm uncomfortably aware that I'm the keynote speaker and I can't be late.

Seeing that the rain is not going to relent, the driver of the van gets out and makes his way around to our sliding back door with a large, sturdy, bright-blue umbrella and escorts us to the building entrance one at a time.

The CARPHA Conference in Grenada is the first Caribbean conference on the built environment and health. CARPHA, the Caribbean Public Health Agency, is an agency backed by its member nations that provides them with supports on public health issues. For the Health and Built Environment workshop, we have convened in a large conference room that takes up the whole of the small, one-story building, and when I enter I'm greeted by colleagues from the Public Health Agency of Canada, who were also asked to attend. Tables have been lined up into a large rectangle in the back two-thirds of the space, and this is where we will be spending our days discussing just what can be done on the different Caribbean islands to improve their built environment for health, with a focus on the epidemics of obesity and their related non-communicable diseases, also a problem in this region. The audience will be local planning and health officials from all over the Caribbean.

I decide to improvise a bit as I start my keynote presentation, throwing in examples from my recent experience of the built environment in Grenada. I explain that I was barely able to cross the street from the hotel to the bus stop to catch my shuttle. There was no traffic light to produce a red for the cars and a green for pedestrians, and though there was a marked crosswalk and a pedestrian crossing light that was supposed to flash to alert the cars to stop, it didn't work. I stood at the edge of the sidewalk for at least ten minutes, making myself and my intention to cross the street as visible as possible, but it was morning rush hour and there were so many cars that I didn't dare try to cross the twenty feet of space. A woman who was trying to catch a local bus at the bus stop bravely made a dash for it, and finally, fearing I would miss my shuttle, I took a deep breath and did the same, running to beat the oncoming traffic from both directions—not an easy feat in a skirt and high-heeled shoes.

I go on to offer my observations about the sidewalks, which are so narrow that people are forced to walk single file. On the busy, narrow road from the hotel to the university, the sidewalks sometimes end abruptly, so that people have no choice but to step onto the road among the speeding cars. It is no wonder, I say, that everyone who can afford to owns one or two cars. It is no wonder that the rate of injuries from motor vehicle and pedestrian collisions is high. It is no wonder that this workshop is so desperately needed here, as elsewhere, in the quickly urbanizing world around us.

Rio de Janeiro is a beautiful city. With a topography of mountains and ocean and beaches in between, it is a city that attracts many international visitors. I'm there for a meeting on my way to

São Paulo, Brazil, where I have been invited to lecture to and advise public health, planning, and architecture professionals on improving health through the built environment.

I arrive in Rio with one of my team members in the middle of the afternoon. The next day, I'll be meeting in the morning with a Columbia University colleague who has been stationed there at one of the university's Global Center offices, now situated in several cities around the world. After checking in, and then hanging my meeting and presentation attire in the hotel room closet, hoping to get out as many wrinkles as possible from being folded in my suitcase for the nine-hour overnight flight from New York, I head down to the hotel lobby. The young woman at the front desk, who tells us that she hopes this job will help improve her English because she wants to pass the entrance exam to the university, recommends a few sights we can take in before dinner. She also instructs us to remove our earrings, to make sure we carry some cash to hand over in case we are robbed, and to stay on the beachfront drive and not wander into the back streets. With that, we enthusiastically, yet nervously, make our way outside to explore the area. We decide, however, to eat dinner at the hotel, since she's also advised us to make our way back to the hotel before dark. "The beach is not safe at night," she warned. Even with all the hotel rooms, like mine, facing the Copacabana beach, it's not enough to keep it safe.

Rio de Janeiro would say it has invested a great deal of money in tourism. It has built a cable car that will take you up its renowned Sugar Loaf Mountain. It has built a train that will take you up to the huge statue, *Christ the Redeemer*, that perches on a mountain overlooking the city. My team member and I visit these sites, lamenting that we can not walk to them, meandering the city's back streets, stopping at locally owned small businesses to eat and to shop. The tourist books, the hotel staff, the locals themselves all warn against such activity. So, instead, we take a Gray Line bus to visit these sites, and we eat lunch at the one restaurant that the tour buses all seem to use for tourists. For other meals, we eat at the restaurants in international hotel chains. I have to ask myself just how much, or rather how little, this form of tourism has benefited local businesses and shop owners. This is so different from New York's Times Square, where all the pedestrians, many of them tourists, have propelled the district and its many stores into one of the top ten retail areas around the world.

Even in cities where incredible work is happening on such fronts as active transportation—cities like Bogotá, Colombia, with its weekly *ciclovía* and its TransMilenio Bus Rapid Transit system— the rapid pace of globalization creates challenges that it will take all our concerted efforts to address. In Bogotá, the introduction of global fast food giants is a recent phenomenon. My health department colleagues there have told me that many people in the city still cook and eat at home—and if they go out, they visit locally owned restaurants that serve traditional Colombian food. But they have observed many in the younger generation beginning to regularly visit the fast food venues.

Although the world does not yet have much experience with using zoning to control the proliferation of fast food and unhealthy food in our cities, towns, and suburbs, I believe we must proceed to do this. We have experience enough using zoning to help prevent our children from being exposed to alcohol retail outlets, for example. But a great deal of our focus in trying to control unhealthy food—both in our discourse and in our actions—has occurred on the national front, particularly with federal agricultural policies and subsidies. Although this is a necessary and essential component of the dialogue and work in policy-making, attempts at national change meet pushback from powerful food industry lobby groups, which means that change is slow at best and very much lacking or thwarted at worst. There is a great need, and opportunity, for cities, towns, and counties that really want to do something about the proliferation of unhealthy food in our neighborhoods—often the neighborhoods with the highest burdens of obesity and diabetes, with children trying their hand at making their own choices without the benefit of their parents' better judgment—to act now to create a healthier balance of choices for their residents. Some cities have begun this work. In addition to Detroit's ban on fast food restaurants in the immediate vicinity of schools, Los Angeles, for example, has put a recent moratorium on new fast food outlets in the areas of their city with the highest numbers of fast food restaurants. Such municipal initiatives, however, are still too few and far between. Even in Detroit, there is a need to expand the area of the fast food ban around schools beyond a mere five hundred feet.

As cities grow, as new neighborhoods are being built and developed, as places like Bogotá globalize with the introduction of the international chains, it is imperative that zoning standards to set a healthier mix of food-related choices—ensuring the existence, or hopefully abundance, of venues offering healthy foods and beverages, and mandating a healthy ratio of healthy to unhealthy food venues and choices—be developed, implemented, and evaluated. We must not allow our new and existing neighborhoods to fall prey to a proliferation of unhealthy choices offered by international chains with deep, deep pockets for building and marketing. We must not accept the loss of local healthy food vendors, who have to struggle to compete. Local governments can begin to define the healthy choices—and the healthy minimum ratio of such choices to unhealthy ones—that must be present in all neighborhoods, so that their residents too can truly make meaningful choices for fitness, for losing or controlling their weight, and for their overall health.

Another key next step, globally, I believe, is training. Not just one-offs, but training that is repeated often enough for a sufficient number of people in the different disciplines needed to achieve environmental change to be trained. With support from the Kresge Foundation and the U.S. Centers for Disease Control and Prevention, such training was created and then offered repeatedly locally and across the U.S. by the New York City health department's Built Environment and Active Design Program. Training can and should be implemented elsewhere for both practicing professionals and professionals in training across various disciplines—health, planning, architecture, housing, transportation. A replication of such successful trainings is needed in different cities to reach people around the world. And also needed are courses that can bring people from cities around the world together.

It is the first week of June 2015, and today is the first day of my Columbia University course Designing Healthy Cities to Reverse Obesity and Non-Communicable Disease Epidemics. After making my way to the course venue—a high-rise building at Columbia's public health and medicine campus way uptown in Manhattan—on a dreary day of wind and rain, I load my overview presentation onto the classroom computer and then wait for my students to arrive. Those who have signed up for the course include university students, university professors, and practicing professionals in urban planning, public health, environmental sustainability, and even journalism. And my students will be local, from New York City, Long Island, and Connecticut, but also from Canada, Brazil, and Taiwan. The course is focused on teaching interested people from different disciplines to take available academic research and the evidence supporting it and apply it in the difficult real-world practice of improving our physical environments for health. It sounded to me like a fun challenge that could make a real difference in the field. Now, I'm working with universities elsewhere, including the University of Alberta in Canada, to create similar courses to reach those who may not be able to travel to New York. And we have been repeating that successful course at Columbia University annually.

There is also something to be said, though, for a course that aims to bring local professionals together to work toward solving their particular local problems. One of my recent trips abroad was to conduct multi-sector training for Macau, China. Macau is a special territory that, like Hong Kong, is exempt from the usual visitor visa requirements of mainland China. This comes as a relief, because several times I've had to spend hours waiting in line for the Chinese consulate, on the far west end of 42nd Street in New York City, to open its doors at 8:00 a.m. in order to get visas for consulting trips to Shanghai and Beijing. This time, all I had to do was email the organizers my training presentation and materials . . . and pack!

This training was a follow-up to a meeting a few years back in Shanghai at which I had been a special adviser to the World Health Organization (WHO) Western Pacific Region Office. The same WHO office was now organizing the training for Macau's Health Bureau. Macau's public health officials had been among the attendees at that Shanghai meeting, and had been intrigued by the presentations that had been given there by myself and by my colleague, Chew Ling, from the Singapore Health Promotion Board. They wanted to learn more about cross-sectoral approaches from me. And they wanted to learn more from the Singapore Health Promotion Board about their government-involved "healthy hawkers' center" initiatives (see chapter 4). As well as local health professionals, the Macau meeting included a small array of other sectors, such as the police. The partnerships weren't yet extensive, but it would be a start to their cross-sectoral work. Since it was a workshop, the participants would be broken up into cross-sectoral teams to brainstorm together and identify their local health priorities and potential locally based solutions.

Such trainings and courses are happening, too, in many North American cities. In Edmonton, Alberta, my old hometown (and now my new hometown, too!) I initiated a cross-sectoral course for the University of Alberta. The university had fairly recently created a School of Urban and Regional Planning, and its inaugural chair, Sandeep Agrawal, had seen my keynote presentation in Fredericton, New Brunswick at the 2014 annual national conference of the Canadian Institute of Planners. On one of the conference's field tours—to see the new pedestrian bridge connecting city neighborhoods on opposite sides of the city's river to the other—we got to talking. Sandeep had also joined an earlier field tour that day that brought him and several others to the site on bicycles. He was in his spandex bicycle shorts, helmet still on, when our discussion began. We talked about the course I had created for Columbia University, and another that I had designed for New York's Pratt Institute. He recognized that he wanted to see just such a course offered through his new department.

And so, in February 2016, urban planning students were brought together with urban planners working in government, health ministry staff with local disease and risk factor data to share, recreation professionals, private sector developers, and even the mayor of the Edmonton suburb of St. Albert, Nolan Crause, and a former St. Albert city councilor, Len Bracko. (St. Albert was coincidentally where my parents first settled in the province, and where my brother and I started our schooling in Canada.) One developer, Greg Christenson of Christenson Developments, gave us a tour of one of his projects: a downtown development that had been designed to foster the revitalization of an area that was largely just abandoned railway lands, a nearly deserted area and desert-like, in need of city water and sanitation connections and other amenities. Greg led the tour and showed us bicycle and walking trails—both a transportation and a recreation amenity—that had been integrated among the development's multiple condo and townhouse buildings, some geared toward seniors, others geared toward luxury downtown living. This had been a rails-to-trails project of sorts too, only starting with new, higher-density housing as the focus. We noted how the trails came to an abrupt end where the private development ended, only a few blocks away from Edmonton's river valley network of parks and recreation trails. If only the different sectors, government and private, had found a way to co-create this initiative along with much-needed surrounding amenities, like bicycle lane connections onto the city's streets. It is my hope that through the training course, the different disciplines and players being brought together will spark just such co-creation projects. And I am happy to report that now, three years later, the bicycle lanes have indeed been painted onto the connecting city streets, and these lanes in turn connect onto yet another off-road bicycle path leading to the miles of trails in the river valley.

Transforming Through Innovation and Technology

Innovations in technology. Innovations in recreation spaces. Innovations in the design of basic amenities. These too are opportunities that we will need to capitalize on, because thus far we have not done so sufficiently. There is a segment—or several segments—of our population that spends significant amounts of time watching sports. While favorite athletes and sports teams exert themselves, getting fitter, burning calories, these fans are sedentary, sprawled on their couches, eating potato chips or nachos. Or sprawled on paid-for seats in an auditorium or sports field, eating hot dogs and french fries. Even parents who have made it their mission to get their children active by signing them up for team sports find themselves sitting for hours on end as they wait for and watch their children practice or compete. Their usual alternatives are to sit on the benches or bleachers, or head to the café to have a hot dog, hamburger, chicken fingers, french fries, or pizza. As their children stay fit, the parents themselves gain weight. Time spent getting their children healthier takes a toll on their health.

Many people have said they have little or no time to exercise. But they would like to, they say. They continue to make their New Year's resolutions. And they continue to fail.

In addition to transforming our neighborhood designs— transformations that will take time, particularly in existing suburban neighborhoods—perhaps we need to think about innovations in our recreation spaces. What if these parents, what if all sports spectators could find a more active way to pass the many hours they usually spend sitting? What if all the seats for watching Little League—or the major leagues—were not just seats? What if there were exercise bikes and elliptical machines that spectators could use at sports venues? What if parents had opportunities for healthy choices while ensuring that their children were active and healthy? What if children could see their parents modeling healthy and active behaviors in adulthood, while they play?

Taipei's parks have done just that. Surrounding their playgrounds and children's play equipment, instead of benches, they have outdoor elliptical machines, exercise bikes, and weight and stretching equipment for adults to use. Some parents and grandparents can be seen sitting on the exercise bikes, pedaling some, resting some. Others spend their whole time on the ellipticals, making good use of their children's play time to get in their own physical activity.

In Hong Kong, a dance club is using innovations in technology to green its space. Energy-capturing floors turn the stomping, jumping, moving feet of its customers into electricity. I have often asked myself: What if all our building hallways, the steps of our stairs, even our sidewalks used such energy-capturing technology? Sure, the technology might need improvement. Sure, it is expensive now. But adoption and use of the technology is precisely what is needed to bring down the cost and identify and fix the glitches.

For ourselves and our children, there are now backpacks that can capture the energy of our movement, of our walking—energy enough to perhaps charge a cell phone. I have charged my own cell phone by plugging it into one of the outdoor exercise bikes on the streets of San Francisco. There are similar charger bikes at Charles de Gaulle Airport in Paris. What if our wish to make our environments greener could be made through our own bodies, through our innovative choices for health? What if more cities made the choice to use the technological innovations available now to motivate their residents and visitors to be healthier and greener all at once?

In Switzerland, there is a hotel whose back side you can ski down, creating an amenity usually associated with a trip to the national park. There is also, in Copenhagen, a residential building called the "8 House," shaped like a figure eight seen from above. Here, front terraces connect to a long, low-grade, sloping ramp that makes its way up and down the figure eight; the ramp passes condo units as it makes its way up from the city's street at the bottom to the top of the building, and then again from the top of the building past more condo units down to the bottom of the building and back to the streets. Residents use the long ramp to ride their bicycles from the street up to their condos at the end of their workday, and then down again to work the next morning. Denmark's pavilion at the Shanghai World Expo also incorporated a ramp, this time one that coiled up a round building. These are just some of the innovations in design that we heard about from the architecture firm BIG—the Bjarke Ingels Group, named for its founder—at our Fit City 6 Conference. Bjarke Ingels, a youthful, energetic young architect, has built the reputation of his firm on innovative, playful, audacious designs. BIG is now constructing its unusually designed buildings all over the world, including projects in New York City. Bjarke has spoken of the new towers his group is building in Lower Manhattan, which twist upward and look as though they are stepped, evoking a sense of stepping up to heaven. Stairs, bicycle paths, ski hills, all on a building—we need more of this!

We need, too, more innovation in design for other basic amenities. It seems that wherever I go, I hear about the obstacles presented by the local weather. When I am in Canadian cities, or other cities and towns with snowy climates, I hear about the snow. "How can people walk and bicycle in the winter?" I am frequently asked. When I am working with clients in Miami, I hear the same concerns about weather, though the conditions are the very opposite. "How can people walk and bicycle in summer?" they ask me. "It's too hot here for such activities." And my response has two parts.

The first part of my answer is that when it comes to snow, operational decisions within cities and towns are critical. Cities and towns can, like Montreal, clear their car lanes, bicycle lanes, and sidewalks of snow with equal priority. If city or town officials are more courageous in their push for health and well-being, greening, and even retail and economic outcomes, they can clear the snow on bicycle lanes and sidewalks first. That's what cities like Copenhagen do, allowing seniors and children as well as adults to use these routes for safe, easy travel throughout the year. Copenhagen is on track to reach its goal of at least 50 percent of its population traveling on city streets—and even suburban streets—on bicycles.

The second part of my answer is that, in order to address weather in the local context, we need innovations in design for the local context. Is there any reason why every bicycle lane must be nothing but a painted lane on the side of a street? Bicycle lanes can be moved from their usual position—precariously in between parked cars and moving vehicles—to a position between the sidewalk and the parked cars, with the parked cars acting as a protector. So, can't bicycle lanes come with other amenities?

Like roofs and awnings, perhaps? If bicycle lanes are more routinely located between city sidewalks and parked cars, then rainy cities can perhaps more easily find ways to shield both their pedestrians and their cyclists to keep them dry. Windy cities might consider more innovative landscaping and design to shield pedestrians and cyclists from the weather. Infrastructure materials matter too, and more can be and should be done to address them. Are there road surfaces that work better for the bicycle? Are there surfaces that work best for pedestrians of different ages and physical abilities and needs? There are now technologies to heat sidewalks so that they may never need to be shoveled . . .

And Also . . . The Social Determinants of Health

"We shouldn't forget the social determinants of health, also," I am telling Jenny Che, a reporter from *The Huffington Post*, who is interviewing me for an article about workplace health. As our interview ends, I emphasize again that organizations really need to support the health of the people who work for them by making healthy choices possible, in both the physical and the social environments that people find themselves in day after day.

Of course, I am thrilled that an increasing number of cities and countries around the world are finding help to improve their physical environments in order to address today's epidemics of obesity and related chronic diseases, and at the same time to also improve their environmental and economic issues. But I also recognize that this isn't enough.

I hope that another new movement may be afoot. A movement that will address persistent issues related to health, issues such as lack of access to good education, or even education at all, for children of families living in poverty; absolute and relative material deprivation arising from low wages and income inequality; and stressful working conditions. And these issues bring me full circle to my early days in medical school, when my interest in public health was piqued by this idea of health having a set of social determinants.

In 1999, I was in my third year of residency in Public Health and Preventive Medicine at the University of Toronto, and much of that year for me was taken up by my work at the Institute for Work and Health, a world-renowned institute for research into work factors and their impacts on health. I was summarizing the research that had been done on sources of work stress and cardiovascular disease. Each morning for nine months of that year I would find myself walking to the St. Clair West subway station from the walk-up apartment that I shared with roommates in one of the few apartment buildings that could be found just east of Spadina Avenue on Lonsdale Road in the Forest Hill area of Toronto. I would take the subway downtown to St. Patrick Station, then walk to a high-rise building at the northeast corner of Dundas Street and University Avenue. When I reached my floor, I would swipe my cardkey and enter the offices of the Institute.

During that time, I had recently completed the Master of Health Science program, and I had learned a great deal about the social determinants of health, including fascinating research evidence showing the impact of the sanitation movement and improvements to the physical environment on improving public health in the nineteenth and early twentieth centuries. I learned, too, the importance of social environments to public health; for example, the education of women is now well known in public health to be an important factor in improving key health indicators such as infant mortality, as well as child health outcomes later in life.

I also learned of the studies conducted by a British epidemiologist, Michael Marmot. Professor Marmot was the lead researcher in what came to be known as the Whitehall Studies. "Whitehall" referred to the offices of the British Civil Service, and the Whitehall

Studies were a series of epidemiologic studies conducted on British civil servants, beginning in the early 1970s. Already by then it was well known that being poor was associated with having unfavorable health outcomes. Marmot, a young researcher, had decided to study British civil servants because he wanted to know whether poverty was associated with poor health outcomes due to absolute or relative deprivation. Marmot reasoned that since no one who worked for the British Civil Service would be in absolute poverty, by undertaking studies of employees within the Civil Service he would be able to begin to determine if relative differences in wealth and social status mattered. And indeed, he found, these relative differences did matter—they mattered a lot.

Marmot's studies showed that, with respect to all health outcomes measured, there was consistently a stepwise gradient that could be found from the highest employment grades to the lowest. Those at the lowest employment levels showed the highest rates of deaths, regardless of the causes studied. Those at the next level up showed the next highest rates, and so on, until you reached the highest employment levels, which showed the lowest rates of deaths and disease. This actually seemed counterintuitive at the time. Since none of the subjects in the studies lived in poverty, it had been expected that perhaps those working at the highest employment levels would show higher rates of conditions like heart disease, caused by the mental stress associated with increased responsibility. But this assumption was proved wrong.

Marmot found that after he factored in all the physical and behavioral risk factors known for heart disease—high blood pressure, smoking, exercise, and so on—he was still unable to account for over 50 percent of the gradients that were seen between the employment levels. At least, not yet.

In 1997, Marmot finally solved some of this puzzle. Repeating his Whitehall Studies, this time he also measured another key factor that had been emerging in the research of the 1970s, '80s, and '90s as being an important one for heart disease: how much control one had over one's job. The studies had been showing that job control appeared to be more consistently associated with the development of heart disease than job demands. The jobs most likely to be associated with the development heart disease were those that had high demands coupled with low job control. So, when Marmot included this factor in his subsequent Whitehall Studies, what did he find? The latest study showed that job control was about as important to the gradients in health as all of the other traditional risk factors combined, with the traditional risk factors combined accounting for about 45 percent of the gradient and job control another 45 percent. Marmot had now shown that he could explain about 90 percent of the employment gradients seen in health, gradients in health that had nothing to do with living in poverty. So, in addition to the absolute material deprivation that living in poverty poses, it would appear that elements in our social environments, such as hierarchy and a sense of control, are really important.

Since the early 1990s, another British researcher, Richard Wilkinson, has been publishing studies specifically focusing on income inequality and health. Unlike Marmot's studies, which focused on government workers in Britain, Wilkinson's studies looked across the world. He used known measures of income inequality and compared the health outcomes of more equal and less equal countries. He found he was able to draw a straight diagonal line across the plotted points on his graph comparing life expectancy to income inequality. As income inequality rose across countries, life expectancy dropped, and all sorts of health and social outcomes—ranging from child health outcomes to crime and mental illness to obesity—also got worse.

Wilkinson and his colleagues have conducted further studies, including those looking at how income inequality can affect people in poor neighborhoods and in wealthy neighborhoods.

His studies found that greater income *equality* benefited the health of people in both wealthy and poor areas. In other words, income inequality is not an issue that only the poor should be concerned about, at least not if we care about improving our health.

Bill de Blasio won the November 2013 mayoral election in New York City by running a campaign based on addressing what he called "a tale of two cities." One, a city of the wealthy and prosperous; the other, a city of the poor.

One of my previous projects as a consultant was with New York City's Regional Plan Association, helping them to integrate health considerations in the development of a Fourth Regional Plan for the New York Metropolitan Region, a region consisting of the many cities, towns, and suburbs surrounding New York City in the three states of New York, New Jersey, and Connecticut. In this work, with funding supports from the Robert Wood Johnson Foundation, we considered the health priorities in the region, and we recognized that if we were going to do something about improving these health outcomes, the physical and social environmental determinants had to be addressed. Income inequality, for example. The New York Metropolitan Region is marked by growing inequality. And it is not only the poor who are getting poorer. The middle class is getting poorer, too. In the New York Metropolitan Region, studies have shown that only the top income quintile enjoyed an increase in median income between 1990 and 2013. The second-highest quintile showed stagnant incomes, while the other three quintiles showed a *decrease* in their incomes. In other words, the trickle-down theory so popular with some did not work, at least not in the context of the New York Metropolitan Region's economic growth. Instead, we saw a trickle-up of wealth, and a growing gap in the incomes of the rich compared to everybody else, something being seen increasingly elsewhere too.

In the New York Metropolitan Region, we also found disparities in educational access. Forty-two percent of Blacks and 40 percent of Hispanics were living in high-poverty neighborhoods, and their children were disproportionately attending schools in poorly performing school districts. With education such an important determinant of health, it is no wonder that the health of these demographic groups is disproportionately poor. The assault of unequally unhealthy physical and social environments on these poor children is leaving its mark permanently on their health.

When Dr. Mary Bassett was appointed Health Commissioner by Mayor de Blasio, I immediately sent her an email asking for a meeting. I wanted to discuss what we could possibly do with the new mayor within the context of the social determinants of health. She accepted, and I prepared for our meeting by undertaking a literature search and drafting a document listing ideas for discussion, a document I would leave behind for her after our meeting.

Our meeting was on a very cold day in early 2014, and I made my way to her midtown Manhattan office, in the high-rise building that housed the Doris Duke Charitable Foundation, where she had until recently been program director for their African Health Initiative. I was shown to her office and found Mary frantically sending emails, clearing her desk, and preparing for a trip to Zimbabwe, after which she would take up her new position at the Department of Health and Mental Hygiene. Mary had previously been a deputy commissioner at the health department when I first started, and I remembered her as someone who cared deeply about social justice. Tall and slim, Mary had a head of dark, curly hair that was just starting to be peppered with gray.

Mary asked about my ideas, and I was only too happy to share them, having waited for years—a decade and a half, in fact, since my residency project on work stress and heart disease—to delve once again into the social determinants of health.

According to the World Health Organization, health has three major determinants:

- the social and economic environment,
- the physical environment, and
- the person's individual characteristics and behaviors.

The above three categories can be broken down further into:

- Income and social status—higher income and social status are linked to better health. The greater the gap between the richest and poorest people, the greater the differences in health.
- Education—low levels of education are linked with poor health, more stress, and lower self-confidence.
- Physical environment—safe water and clean air, healthy workplaces, safe houses, communities, and roads all contribute to good health.
- Employment and working conditions—people in employment are healthier, particularly those who have more control over their working conditions.
- Social support networks—greater support from families, friends, and communities is linked to better health.
- Culture—customs and traditions, and the beliefs of the family and community all affect health.
- Genetics—inheritance plays a part in determining lifespan, healthiness, and the likelihood of developing certain illnesses.
- Personal behavior and coping skills—balanced eating, keeping active, not smoking, not drinking inappropriately, and how we deal with life's stresses and challenges all affect health.

- Health services—access to and use of services that prevent and treat disease influence health.
- Gender—men and women suffer from different types of diseases at different ages.

The World Health Organization defines the "social determinants of health" as "the conditions in which people are born, grow, work, live, and age, and the wider set of forces and systems shaping the conditions of daily life. These forces and systems include economic policies and systems, development agendas, social norms, social policies and political systems."

Other organizations have also attempted to quantify the impacts of the different determinants. In the United States, the Robert Wood Johnson Foundation has worked with the University of Wisconsin to quantify the different factors contributing to health. While clinical care contributes about 20 percent, physical environmental factors and health opportunities together contribute about 40 percent, and social and economic factors— like education, employment, income, family and social support, and community safety—are thought to contribute the final 40 percent.

In my work with the Regional Plan Association, we created an adaptation of this model of the determinants of health for urban planning. In this adaptation, we showed that the physical environment can shape not only water and air quality, but the opportunities for health-related behaviors, behaviors like tobacco use, diet and exercise, and alcohol and drug use. We started to show also how the physical environment can additionally shape the social and economic environment. Housing policies are particularly important.

In 2014, I wrote a paper for the World Health Organization entitled "Working Across Sectors for Health Equity" for their special report *Cities for Health*. In this paper, I discussed the possibility of improving the physical environment and standards for the physical environment across all neighborhoods, including and especially impoverished neighborhoods, as one critical way to address the health disparities so often seen in our cities. But in my recent work with the New York City Metropolitan Area's Fourth Regional Plan, I have also been advocating for increased consideration and action on the interplay of our physical and social environmental factors. We can shape even educational access with the choices that we make concerning housing. Yes, really. If we have only large, expensive, single-family homes in good school districts, then only wealthy children will have access to those schools. If we have only poorly designed low-cost apartment rentals in poor school districts, then the local tax base formula used in the United States to fund schools means that those school districts will never be able to improve. So, our housing mix policies—our built environment policies—and whether they integrate a range of incomes in all our communities are also drivers of the social environments of different neighborhoods and consequently affect health outcomes.

But the social and economic environments that are *not* shaped by the physical environment also need to be addressed.

Mary Bassett has implemented some of the ideas we discussed together—for example, creating a new office within the New York City Department of Health and Mental Hygiene with a focus on health equity—but there is a great deal more to do. I have suggested that the city, under its current administration, could become an example of what is possible in terms of making interventions to positively affect the critical social environmental determinants, just as we showed what was possible in making changes to physical environmental determinants under Mayor Bloomberg. Why not use City of New York government projects and workplaces to show what can be done? With Mayor de Blasio having emphasized income inequality—the "tale of two cities"—as his main campaign platform, I suggested that the City set an explicit maximum income gap, even if not initially for the union-ized employees, then for its non-union employees. We can do this in Canada also, for example, starting with the income poli-cies found in public health and health care organizations and the government sector. I suspect that in the public sector it would in fact be very feasible to set a relatively narrow income gap, since the existing differential between top and bottom pay scales is unlikely to be of the width seen in the private sector. In the U.S. private sector, there is, on average, an over-300-fold difference, which can stretch to an over-1,000-fold difference, between CEO and worker salaries. I am still waiting to see this happen in the public sector in New York, and I find myself asking: If not under the administration that won an election based on its commit-ment to ending income inequality, then when?

For those who believe that there should be no limits on income when it recognizes talent and results? A fixed income gap is not a fixed maximum income. Rather, it's a policy that would allow everyone in a company to feel motivated toward growth, because company outcomes that bring the CEO and top executives bonuses and higher salaries would mean bonuses and higher salaries for everyone else in the company, too. I believe in our unlimited potential—and I believe in fairness, and in being equally motivat-ing to all of a company's employees.

There is much talk of minimum wages these days, but much less talk about what can be done to address income inequality. However, in the United States, as in Canada, after years of stag-nant minimum wages, there is now a reconsideration of these wages that can leave even full-time workers and their families in poverty. Even in 1997, when I was studying for my master's degree at the University of Toronto, minimum wage had fallen so far behind the initial 1970s levels that a person earning a minimum hourly wage would have to work over seventy hours a week to reach the poverty threshold set by Statistics Canada. Fortunately, there are initiatives now that are raising, or planning to raise, Canadian and American minimum wages. But these discussions must ensure that indexing for inflation is built in, so that any new progress made isn't soon lost again to inflation.

As I sit with the reporter from *The Huffington Post*, I find I must also share with her some additional ideas that I have for these social determinants of health. I tell her I think responsible companies, and even government employers, can start to set standards for a maximum income gap. We could opt for a maximum six- or ten- or even twenty-fold difference in the ratio of top to bottom salaries and a maximum ratio too for top to average salaries in our organizations. It is not unheard of. Though the situation may be changing more recently, Japan has had gaps in the range of a six-fold difference between CEO and worker salaries. Japan, I tell her, has today's longest life expectancy and lowest per-capita health care spending.

I tell her about job control. "Employers don't have to wait for their employees to take a stress management course, courses that many employees don't take up even when offered, probably because they have to rush home to their kids after work," I tell her. There are things employers can start to do now. They can directly structure their workplace social environments to give their employees more control over their jobs, wherever and whenever that is appropriate. So, while someone sitting at the front desk might not be able to work from 9:00 a.m. to 5:00 p.m., if a business is open from 8:00 a.m. to 4:00 p.m., perhaps the person sitting in the back office can if that is the needed flexibility that makes the difference between more work-life balance rather than less. If there are multiple front desk staff, perhaps there is some way to stagger their schedules according to their needs rather than using a system that sets those schedules arbitrarily. There are many other strategies. Some cities in Europe have restructured bus routes and schedules with the help of their drivers to more realistically achieve the scheduled stops, to increase a sense of control for the drivers, and to drive down their high rates of heart disease.

And again, fundamentally, I find myself talking about the creation of more choices. In the social sphere, as it is in the physical environment, helping people to be healthy, to be more fit, is fundamentally about what our governments and our organizations can do to give people more choices. Choices shape our health—whether we are choosing how best to structure our seven- or eight-hour work day so it balances our family's needs, or choosing what we buy because we have a non-poverty-level wage, or choosing to work harder or less hard because company outcomes ultimately shape our incomes as well as our CEO's, or choosing to eat healthy food or drink water because it is available to be chosen, or choosing to walk or bike to work.

When we can make these choices ourselves, we are taking control of our health. And a key role of fit cities is to facilitate such choices, to make them choices that are truly possible for people.

ACKNOWLEDGEMENTS

Many thanks to Linda Pruessen for her invaluable assistance in helping me tell my story.

Lynn Henry at Penguin Random House Canada was the very first person to believe in this book. Thank you, Lynn, for creating this wonderful opportunity. And thanks to Bonnie Henry, an incredibly dedicated public health physician, for connecting me in the first place to Lynn.

At Doubleday Canada, multiple other people then supported and guided me throughout the writing, editing, and publication process with their depth and breadth of experience. Thank you especially to Amy Black and Tim Rostron. Thank you also to copy editor Catherine Marjoribanks for her further refinements. I would like to thank my agent, Trena White, for her ever-helpful guidance.

I am also grateful to my colleagues from around the world whose efforts and collaborations have contributed to the gains made to date in obesity and non-communicable disease prevention and control. Many of them are mentioned within the book.

I also want to thank the wonderful faculty and staff with whom I now work daily and whose ideas, encouragement, and partnerships help to fuel my continued enthusiasm and efforts for all the work that remains to be done.

I also want to call out my very insufficient thanks to the people whose love, support, and belief in me have made this book, as well as so many other accomplishments and joys in my life, possible: Anne Lee and Andrew Lee; Mark Lee and Jennifer Stickney-Lee; Matthew Lee and Rebecca Lee; Pat, Jim, and Alysa Englehardt; Long Litt Woon; Drs. Anna Bendzsak; Nadia Khan; Helen Kwon; Shanu Modi; Randy Staab; and Vanessa Wong. Also, Cheri Blain; Shoela Detsios; Fiona English; Pearl Goodman; Todd Graham; Rose Lee; Denise Yap; Helen Yoon and Davide Rossi; Vanessa Cosco and David Woo; Brent Windwick and Brenda Kaminski; and James Mallet and Sarah Thomsen. Thank you all for being a part of my life and for enriching it and its many adventures.

NOTES ON SOURCES

As those who have written peer-review scientific journal publications know, sometimes the list of citations for references can well exceed even the length of the paper itself.

For the purposes of this book, intended for the general reader as well as specialists, I've taken the approach of citing broader databases and sources that house more detailed references.

Resources that I have been personally involved in developing can be found on the "Resources," "Projects," and "News" pages at http://www.drkarenlee.com. See also the references cited in these sources.

For additional scientific publications, readers can go to "PubMed" at https://www.ncbi.nlm.nih.gov/m/pubmed/ and search by author(s) and/or key topics. For example, for studies by Richard Wilkinson on income inequality, one can go to PubMed and search "Wilkinson R income inequality." The latest review articles often provide helpful summaries of the overall evidence. Review articles can be searched by topic plus "review article." For example, for review articles on the links between supermarket initiatives and nutrition outcomes, search by using the key words "supermarket nutrition review article."

Another good source of scientific reviews is The Community Guide, which can be accessed at https://www.thecommunityguide.org.

Scientific reviews that have been completed by the U.S. Task Force on Community Preventive Services (convened by the U.S. Department of Health and Human Services) can also be searched by topic plus your area of interest. For example, selecting "physical activity" pulls up a list of interventions that have been tried within various community settings, along with information about when the review was completed by the task force and whether the intervention reviewed had strong evidence, sufficient evidence, or insufficient evidence at the time of the review.

Note that although scientific reviews help to capture the state of the evidence overall, the most recent or emerging scientific evidence may be missed in a review if a recent primary study was published or conducted after the review was completed. Initiatives may also not yet have been the subject of review articles if they are very new or there have not been enough studies done on them in order to complete a review.

In addition to PubMed, other sources of active living and healthy eating studies include Active Living Research and Healthy Eating Research, which can be found respectively at https://activelivingresearch.org and https://healthyeatingresearch.org.

Sources for statistics on trends and prevalence of diseases and risk factors include PubMed publications, World Health Organization reports (https://www.who.int/news-room/fact-sheets/detail/noncommunicable-diseases), the U.S. Centers for Disease Control and Prevention (https://www.cdc.gov), and Statistics Canada (https://www.statcan.gc.ca).